The
EVERYTHING®
Pregnancy Book

Dear Reader:

When I was pregnant with my first child, I was overwhelmed by the sheer volume of pregnancy and childbirth information available, and completely underwhelmed by the available means to sort through it all. Everyone had advice for me, usually some unsolicited nugget of wisdom passed along from her neighbor's third cousin. Although my health care providers were wonderful, they weren't able to answer those 2 A.M. "was that a kick or heartburn?" questions, nor were they able to address more practical matters such as negotiating more maternity leave or finding clothing that didn't look like it was from the Gymboree plus-size collection. In that spirit, I hope you find this book, *The Everything® Pregnancy Book, Second Edition,* to be useful as a survival manual to get you through this next 9 months.

So, congratulations to you and your family for embarking on this grand adventure. As you adjust to the idea of becoming a mom (or a repeat mom), and start to get to know that little person growing inside you, make sure you take time to savor your pregnancy. Nine months may seem like a long time, but to prepare for a lifetime of parenthood it's merely a weekend seminar.

Sincerely,

Paula Ford-Martin

D1405051

THE
EVERYTHING®
PREGNANCY
BOOK

SECOND EDITION

What every woman needs to know—
month-by-month—to ensure a worry-free pregnancy

Paula Ford-Martin with
Elisabeth A. Aron, M.D., F.A.C.O.G.

Adams Media Corporation
Avon, Massachusetts

For Cassie and Kate, both well worth the wait.

An Everything® Series Book.
Everything® and everything.com® are registered trademarks of F+W Publications, Inc.

Published by Adams Media, an F+W Publications Company
57 Littlefield Street, Avon, MA 02322 U.S.A.
www.adamsmedia.com

ISBN: 1-58062-808-7
Printed in the United States of America.

J   I   H   G   F   E   D   C   B

Library of Congress Cataloging-in-Publication Data
Ford-Martin, Paula.
The everything pregnancy book / Paula Ford-Martin,
with Elisabeth A. Aron.– 2nd ed.
p.   cm.   (An everything series book)
Rev. ed. of: The everything pregnancy book /
Maryann Brinley and Stephanie Goldpin. 1999.
ISBN 1-58062-808-7
1. Pregnancy–Popular works. 2. Childbirth–Popular works.
[DNLM: 1. Pregnancy–Popular Works. WQ 150 F711e 2003] I. Aron,
Elisabeth A. II. Brinley, Maryann Bucknum. Everything pregnancy book.
III. Title. IV. Series: Everything series.
RG525.B666   2003
618.2'4–dc21   2003004471

This book is available at quantity discounts for bulk purchases.
For information, call 1-800-872-5627.

Contents

Acknowledgments / ix
Top Ten Things Every Pregnant Woman Should Know / x
Introduction / xi

Getting Ready / 1
So You're Pregnant . . . **2** • A Different Kind of Family Tree **2** • Finding a Health Care Provider **3** • Smoking Cessation **9** • Avoiding Alcohol **10** • Eating Right **11** • Exercising Your Body **15** • Using Medications and Supplements **16** • On Your Mind **18** • Genetic Counseling **19** • Chronic Health Conditions **21**

Month 1 / 23
Baby This Month **24** • Your Body This Month **25** • At the Doctor **28** • On Your Mind **33** • Morning Sickness **34** • Just for Dads **38**

Family Matters / 39
Make Room for Baby **40** • The High Cost of Having a Baby **45** • Financial Planning for a Bigger Family **48** • Lifestyle Changes, or Stating the Obvious **51** • Sharing Pregnancy with the Dad-to-Be **51** • Single Moms and Support **52** • An Eye Toward the Future **53**

Month 2 / 55
Baby This Month **56** • Your Body This Month **58** • At the Doctor **59** • On Your Mind **60** • Dressing for Two **62** • Just for Dads **64**

Diagnostic Tests and Screening / 67
The Basics **68** • Urine Tests **68** • Blood Work **71** • Swabs and Smears **74** • Ultrasounds **75** • Alpha-fetoprotein (AFP)/Triple or Quad Screen Test **78** • Amniocentesis **79** • Chorionic Villus Sampling (CVS) **81** • Fetal Monitoring **82** • Biophysical Profile (BPP) **84**

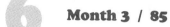
6

Month 3 / 85

Baby This Month **86** • Your Body This Month **86** • At the Doctor **90** • On Your Mind **91** • Spreading the Word **93** • Just for Dads **95**

7

Multiple Choice: Two, Three, Four, or More / 97

Splitting Eggs and Sharing Sacs **98** • Who Has Multiples? **99** • Your Body in Multiples Pregnancy **100** • Doctor's Visits **101** • Problems in Multiple Pregnancies **102** • Delivering Multiples **106** • Surviving the First Month Home **108**

8

Month 4 / 113

Baby This Month **114** • Your Body This Month **115** • At the Doctor **119** • On Your Mind **119** • Exercise **120** • Just for Dads **123**

9

Working Through Pregnancy / 125

Your Rights **126** • Occupational Hazards **128** • Breaking the News **128** • Avoiding the "Mommy-Track" Trap **129** • Practical Matters **132** • Maternity Leave **134** • Back to Work **136** • Changing Paths **137**

10

Month 5 / 141

Baby This Month **142** • Your Body This Month **143** • At the Doctor **147** • On Your Mind **148** • Sleeping Tight **149** • Just for Dads **152**

11

Repeat Performance: Second or Subsequent Pregnancies / 155

Baby and Your Body **156** • Sharing the News **158** • On Your Child's Mind **159** • Involving the Sibling(s)-to-Be **162** • The Second-Time Father **163** • Living Large: When You Choose a Big Family **164**

12

Month 6 / 167
Baby This Month **168** • Your Body This Month **169** • At the Doctor **172** • On Your Mind **172** • Enjoying Your Pregnancy **173** • Just for Dads **175**

13

Special Concerns in Pregnancy / 179
Chronic Illness and High-Risk Pregnancies **180** • Genetic Testing/ Counseling **180** • Ectopic Pregnancy **181** • Molar Pregnancy **182** • Gestational Diabetes **184** • Hyperemesis Gravidarum **187** • Incompetent Cervix **187** • Intrauterine Growth Restriction (IUGR) **188** • Placenta Problems **190** • Preeclampsia/Toxemia/Eclampsia **193** • Premature Labor **194** • Preterm Premature Rupture of Membranes (PPROM) **196** • Bed Rest **196** • Miscarriage **198**

14

Month 7 / 201
Baby This Month **202** • Your Body This Month **203** • At the Doctor **205** • On Your Mind **206** • Childbirth Classes **207** • Just for Dads **212**

15

Blueprint for Birth: Writing Your Birth Plan / 215
Why Have a Birth Plan? **216** • Atmosphere **218** • Family, Friends, and Support **219** • Getting Ready **220** • Pain Relief **222** • When to Change Course: Interventions **223** • Other Considerations **224** • Rooming In or Out **225** • Postpartum Planning **226**

16

Month 8 / 227
Baby This Month **228** • Your Body This Month **229** • At the Doctor **231** • On Your Mind **233** • Nesting **235** • Just for Dads **236**

17

Month 9 / 239
Baby This Month **240** • Your Body This Month **241** • At the Doctor **242** • On Your Mind **243** • Gearing Up for the Big Event **245** • Just for Dads **249**

18   Labor and Delivery / 251

Get Ready: Baby and Your Body in Labor **252** • Get Set: Pain Relief Options **254** • Go! Labor in Three Acts **257** • Caesarean Section **262** • Induction **265** • After Birth **266** • On Your Mind **270** • Just for Dads **270** • The Best Laid Plans **272**

19   Breastfeeding Basics / 275

Breast or Bottle? **276** • Your Body and Breastfeeding **279** • Baby's Body and Breastfeeding **285** • Bottle Basics **286** • Eating Right: For Mom **289** • On Your Mind **290** • Lactation Problems **291** • Just for Dads **295**

20   Bringing Baby Home / 297

Your Body Postpartum **298** • Recovering after Caesarean **299** • Baby's Body: An Operator's Manual **300** • From Soft Spot to Curled Toes **301** • Sleeping Like a Baby **304** • Postpartum Depression **305** • Adjusting to Your New Schedule **307** • The Rest of the Family **309** • Just for Dads **311**

21   Back in the Swing of Things / 313

Getting Your Body Back **314** • The Incredible Changing Baby **317** • Your Career **318** • A Whole New Family **320** • Just for Dads **322**

Appendix A • Additional Resources / **323**

Appendix B • Birth Plan Checklist / **333**

Appendix C • Estimated Due Date Table / **337**

Appendix D • The Practical Side of Pregnancy—A 9-Month Checklist / **341**

Index / 345

Acknowledgments

A special "thank you" to Dr. Elisabeth Aron for lending her perspective and expertise to this book, and to Barb Doyen and Eric M. Hall for their patience, encouragement, and guidance.

I'd also like to acknowledge the contributions and assistance of those women who offered their professional expertise and guidance to the writing of this book, including: Robin Elise Weiss, B.A., L.C.C.E., I.C.C.E.-C.P.E., C.D. (D.O.N.A.)—woman of many acronyms, mother of five, and doula extraordinaire—who was kind enough to share her wisdom on the special role of the doula in the birth experience; Dr. Melissa Stöppler, whose stress management advice was invaluable on a personal as well as a professional level; patient advocate and bestselling author Mary Shomon, who was a wealth of information on postpartum thyroid issues; and adoption advocate Nancy Ashe, who took the time to explain the intricacies of adoption law and birth records to me.

Top Ten Things
Every Pregnant Woman Should Know

1. Morning sickness doesn't just happen in the morning.

2. Alcohol and tobacco in any amount in pregnancy can have serious health repercussions for your baby.

3. Taking 400 micrograms of folic acid before and in early pregnancy can dramatically reduce your risk of having a baby with neural tube defects.

4. Trust your instincts—what worked for your neighbor, friend, or sister isn't necessarily what's right for you.

5. A birth plan can help you and your partner work toward the labor and delivery experience you want.

6. Things don't always go according to plan, but being prepared for the possibilities can make the detours easier to handle.

7. A due date is a suggestion, not a contractual obligation.

8. Career and family are not mutually exclusive.

9. Federal legislation provides specific protections against pregnancy discrimination in the workplace.

10. Stress can be hard on the health of you and your baby; make sure you have a support system for both pregnancy and new motherhood.

Introduction

▶ YOUR MOTHER ALWAYS SAID, "You'll understand when you have kids of your own." And as much as you may hate to admit it, she's right. Being a mom starts the day you find out you're no longer a solo act; suddenly responsibility means more than remembering when the cat needs shots and getting the oil changed every 3,000 miles. Pregnancy initiates you into an empathetic sisterhood of women who can be a source of inspiration, support, and advice throughout pregnancy and beyond.

It's a big club—over four million American women gave birth in 2001—but it's surprisingly intimate in its knowledge of the trials and tribulations of motherhood. Never again will you roll your eyes at a toddler throwing a tantrum in the grocery store, or tap your fingers impatiently at that woman taking forever to load up her kids in the car and pull out of "your" parking space. Mothers understand that pregnancy and parenting takes patience, love, and compassion.

Pregnancy also means preparing for a whole new lifestyle. You and your significant other will no longer be couples-only; your free time will focus on parks and playgroups rather than dinner and a show. If you have children already, the challenges and joys of new sibling relationships are ahead. And your husband or partner will be exploring his new role as a dad and learning the ropes of child care. It's an exciting time, but as with any unfamiliar venture, pregnancy and the prospect of this completely dependent tiny person can inspire anxiety and, yes, even fear. Are you eating the right foods? Is your morning run bad for your baby? Will your child develop your grandfather's diabetes? In true motherly style, you've started worrying about your baby's well-being already.

Of course, your health care provider is the best source of information for specific medical questions about your pregnancy. But even the most dedicated doctor can't be at your disposal 24-7. *The Everything®Pregnancy Book, Second Edition,* was designed as your personal pregnancy assistant—an essential educational reference for your pregnancy concerns and a guide for the more practical matters of career considerations, car seats, and family budgets. It's also a great resource for helping you plan a birth experience you'll treasure.

Most important, this book encourages an open dialogue with your health care provider. Your doctor or midwife can provide medical care and expert advice, but ultimately you must manage your health care for yourself. That means reading up, asking questions, and making sure you're satisfied with the answers. After all, you wouldn't let your financial planner do whatever he pleases with your money without providing some input and approval. Yet many women don't feel they have a right to "bother" their doctors with their questions about a much more precious investment—their child.

You'll make many critical decisions throughout your pregnancy, from pursuing diagnostic testing and genetic counseling to your labor and delivery preferences. Educating yourself allows you to make informed choices and to make the most of your time with your doctor or midwife. Most health care providers are more than willing to answer your questions; patients who do their homework demonstrate their commitment to a healthy pregnancy and make their provider's job easier in the long run. But remember, communication is key. Your questions *will* go unanswered if you fail to ask them.

Enjoy this special time, and consider *The Everything® Pregnancy Book, Second Edition,* a key part of your support team. The highly-coveted "mother's intuition" is usually made, not born, and will come in time as you become better acquainted with your growing baby and learn more about this exciting journey called pregnancy and parenthood. Ⓔ

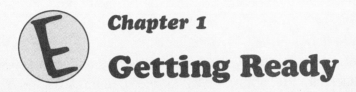

Chapter 1

Getting Ready

Pregnancy is a time of big changes for your family, your body, and your emotional equilibrium. Finding balance, keeping yourself healthy, and choosing a health care provider who will support you in this journey are crucial to creating the best possible environment for baby, both in and out of the womb.

So You're Pregnant . . .

You just found out you're pregnant. Perhaps you've been trying for just a few months, or maybe for a few years. There's also a good chance this baby has taken you by surprise; about half of all pregnancies among American women are unintended. Planned or unplanned, pregnancy stirs up a wide spectrum of emotions. You may be on cloud nine and picking out nursery patterns, or you may be in a state of shock wondering how you're going to handle it all.

Relax. You're normal. Everyone reacts to the joys and jeopardies of pregnancy differently. Preparing yourself for the road ahead is the best way to overcome your fears and get a realistic picture of what pregnancy, and motherhood, is made of. So ask questions, read up, take classes, and talk to friends and family who have been there. There's no such thing as too much information when it comes to your (and your baby's) health.

A Different Kind of Family Tree

Even if you and your partner are the poster people of perfect health, you may have a history of chronic illness or medical disorders further back in your lineage that could impact the health of your unborn child. Your health care provider will ask you questions about your ethnic and racial heritage and family background (and that of the baby's father) to screen for medical conditions your child may be at risk for. Having the most complete and accurate information possible will help her determine what screening tests, if any, you may wish to consider.

In addition to the medical history of you and your partner, as well as any children you already have, you should gather known health information for an additional two generations back (i.e., your parents and siblings and those of your partner, and your second-degree relatives including grandparents, aunts, and uncles). Any additional information you have about medical conditions further back in your family tree should also be brought to your provider's attention.

Parents-to-be who were adopted may have little to no information on their birth families. As of early 2002, only four states (Alabama, Alaska, Kansas, and Oregon) provided open and unconditional access of original birth certificates to all adopted adults; other states provide access with consent of the birth parent or by court order only. If you'd like to pursue access to your health history, your first step is to know the law. Some states allow non-identifying (non-ID) information to be given out. Non-ID is information about the adoption, excluding any information that would enable you to identify the people involved. In many cases, the non-ID information will include some medical and social history of the birth parents, but in some states it is only voluntary and may not be available.

If you have a history of health problems or miscarriage and your doctor feels more family background would be valuable, many states provide a system by which an adoptee can petition the court to get adoption records opened or unsealed.

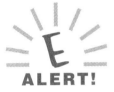

ALERT!

Don't rely too much on the health histories in adoption records. There are no guarantees that the healthy 20-year-old who gave birth didn't develop major medical problems later in life. In many cases, the original adoption information may not even include any medical history beyond a brief physical indicator at the time of the adoption (i.e., "appeared to be in good health").

If you uncover a history of medical problems in your family you were unaware of, keep in mind that only 3 percent of American infants are born with a birth defect, and only a portion of those are thought to have a genetic component. In many cases of inherited diseases, a complex interaction of both genetic and environmental factors is required to trigger the condition. If your provider determines you are at risk for passing along a medical problem to your child, she may refer you to a genetic counselor for further analysis of your risk factors and a discussion of options for additional testing or another appropriate course of action.

Finding a Health Care Provider

Even if you have a picture-perfect pregnancy, you will be seeing a lot of your health care provider over the next 9 months. The American College of Obstetrics and Gynecology (ACOG) recommends that women see their provider every 4 weeks through the first 28 weeks of pregnancy (about 7 months). After 28 weeks, the visits will increase to once every 2 to 3 weeks; after 36 weeks, you'll be paying your doctor or midwife a weekly visit until your baby arrives. If you have any conditions that put you in a high-risk category (e.g., diabetes, history of preterm labor), your provider may want to see you more frequently to monitor your progress.

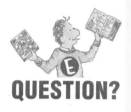

QUESTION?

What is a doula, and is it too early to get one?
A doula is a pregnancy and birth support person, whose job is to provide emotional assistance to both the mom-to-be and her family. Doulas can assist you at any point in pregnancy, from preconception to postpartum. Because doulas tend to work with a variety of physicians and midwives in many different settings, they may also be helpful in providing information on places and providers as you plan your birth experience. (For more on doulas, see Chapter 15.)

The Options

So who should guide you on this odyssey? If you currently see a gynecologist or family practice doctor who also has an obstetric practice, he or she may be a good choice. If you don't have that choice, or would like to explore your options, consider:

- **An ob-gyn**: An obstetrician and gynecologist is a medical doctor (MD) who has received specialized training in women's health and reproductive medicine.
- **A perinatologist**: If you have a chronic health condition, you may see a perinatologist—an ob-gyn who specializes in overseeing high-risk pregnancies.
- **A midwife**: Certified nurse-midwives are licensed to practice in all fifty states. They provide patient-focused care throughout pregnancy, labor, and delivery.
- **Nurse practitioner**: A nurse practitioner is a registered nurse (RN) with advanced medical education and training (at minimum, a Master's degree).

- **Combined practice**: Some obstetrical practices blend midwives, NPs, and MDs, with the choice (or sometimes the requirement) of seeing one or more throughout your pregnancy.

Networking and Referrals

Finding Dr. Right may seem like a monumental task; after all, this is the person you're entrusting your pregnancy and your child with. Unless you're paying completely out-of-pocket for all prenatal care, labor, and delivery expenses, your first consideration is probably your health insurance coverage. If you are part of a managed care organization, your insurer may require that you see someone within their provider network. Getting a current copy of the network directory, if one is available, can help you narrow down your choices by coverage and location.

Many women choose a physician solely for logistical reasons (e.g., insurance will cover all of his fees, or she's nearby work). While money and convenience are important, they won't mean much if you aren't happy with the care you receive and the role you ultimately play in your pregnancy and birth. Whether it's your first or your fifth, this pregnancy is a one-time-only performance. You deserve the best support in seeing it through. Talk to the experts—girlfriends and other women you know and trust—and get referrals. Be aware that not everyone looks for the same thing in a health care provider; what one woman loves you may cringe at. With this in mind, you may find it more efficient to limit your survey to friends and family you know well rather than canvassing your office or gym (as word spreads you'll be getting unsolicited recommendations from your manicurist's daughter's sister-in-law).

If you've just moved to a new area or simply don't know any moms or moms-to-be, there are other referral options available. The licensing authority in your area (the state or county medical board) can typically provide you with references for local practitioners. You may also try the patient services department or labor and delivery programs of nearby hospitals and/or birthing centers. Most medical centers will be happy to offer you several provider referrals, and you can get information on their facilities in the process.

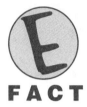

FACT

Need a referral? The American College of Obstetricians and Gynecologists (ACOG) can help. Contact their resource center at ✉409 12th Street, SW, PO Box 96920, Washington, DC 20090-6920, or visit the ACOG online physician referral database at ✐ *www.acog.org* (all ACOG fellows are board certified ob-gyns). To find a nurse-midwife, contact the American College of Nurse Midwives at ✆202-728-9860, or search their midwife listings at ✐ *www.midwife.org*.

Ask the Right Questions

Once you've collected names and numbers and narrowed down your list of potential providers, and have verified that they accept (and are accepted by) your health insurance plan, it's time to do some legwork. Sit down with your partner and talk about your biggest questions, concerns, and expectations. Then, compile a list of "interview questions." Some issues to consider:

- **What are the costs and payment options?** If your health plan doesn't provide full coverage, find out how much the remaining fees will run and if installment plans are available.
- **Who will deliver my baby?** Will the doctor or midwife you select deliver your child, or will it be another provider in the practice depending on when the baby arrives? If your provider works alone, find out who covers his patients during vacations and emergencies.
- **Who will I see during office visits?** Group practices typically share delivery responsibilities, so you may want to ask about rotating your prenatal appointments among all the providers in the group so you'll see a familiar face in the delivery room when the big day arrives.
- **What is your philosophy on routine IVs, episiotomies, labor induction, pain relief, and other interventions in the birth process?** If you have certain expectations regarding medical interventions during labor and delivery, you should lay them out now.
- **What hospital or birthing center will I go to?** Find out where the provider has hospital privileges, and more information on that facility's

programs and policies, if possible. Is a neonatal unit available if problems arise after the baby's birth? Many hospitals offer tours of their labor and delivery rooms for expectant parents.

- **What is your policy on birth plans?** Will the provider work with you to create and, more importantly, follow a birth plan? Will the plan be signed and become part of your permanent chart in case he or she is off-duty during the birth? (For more on birth plans, see Chapter 15 and Appendix B.)
- **How are phone calls handled if I have a health concern or question?** Most obstetrical practices have some sort of triage (or prioritizing) system in place for patient phone calls. Find out how quickly calls are returned and if your provider will be available to speak to if necessary. And since babies don't keep bankers' hours, find out what system they have in place for handling night and weekend patient calls.

Some providers have the staff to answer these sorts of inquiries over the phone, whereas others might schedule a face-to-face appointment with the doctor or midwife you are considering. Either way, make sure that all your questions are answered to your satisfaction so you can make a fully informed choice.

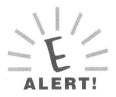

ALERT!

When you phone potential providers, pay close attention to how the support staff handles your call. If the receptionist is rushed or rude, or if you're put on perpetual hold, it may be a sign that the office is understaffed. Midwife and obstetric practices are notoriously busy, but a competent office staff will be both polite and reasonably timely with patient inquiries.

Comfort and Communication

Like any good relationship, communication is essential for patients and their providers. Does she encourage your questions, answer them thoroughly, and really listen to your concerns? Does he make sure all your questions are answered before concluding the appointment? Is the nursing and administrative staff attentive to patients' needs and willing to answer questions as well?

Good health care is a partnership, or more accurately, a team effort. Ultimately, you call the shots (it's your body and baby, after all), but your provider is there as your coach and trainer, giving you the support and training you need to reach that finish line. If your doctor doesn't listen to your needs, she won't be able to meet them. Remember that communication works both ways, as well. Your provider has likely been around the block a few times and has a wealth of useful information to offer you, particularly if you're a rookie at this baby game.

Although experience, education, and practice philosophy are key considerations in selecting a care provider, your comfort is equally important. Is the doctor warm and compassionate, cold and humorless, outgoing and chatty, or reserved and distant? Even with a short introductory phone call or appointment, you should be able to get some feel for your potential provider's bedside manner. Is it a personality style you can effectively deal with for the next 9 months? If you're regaled with bad jokes or mind-numbingly boring clinical explanations at the doctor's office, just imagine how you'll feel hearing it in the delivery room.

Gender may also be an issue for you. Some women feel more at ease with a female physician. Making an issue of gender may seem silly or at worst, discriminatory and hypocritical. The subject is serious enough to merit a number of clinical studies and patient surveys in the medical literature both for and against a clear gender preference. Some reasons given for choosing a woman doctor include communication style and the fact that the physician may have been through pregnancy herself. Other women may find that they prefer a male doctor for various reasons. The bottom line is that you are the one who has to live with your provider choice for the next 9 months, and to spend it feeling awkward, stressed, and inhibited—emotions that can ultimately have a negative effect on your pregnancy—is not healthy. Whatever your choice, make sure it's one you'll be comfortable with.

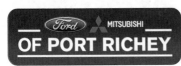
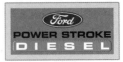

Wholesale Parts Direct: 888-351-1695
Service & Sales: 727-868-9545

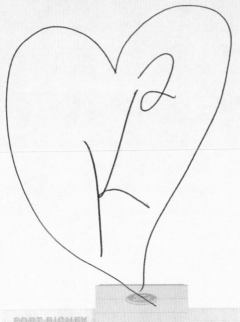

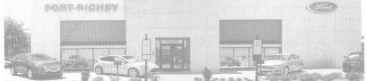

Smoking Cessation

The life inside you is dependent on your "delivery system" for its very existence. Taking care of yourself—body and mind—over these next 9 months will be your number-one priority for raising a healthy baby.

You don't need anyone to tell you that cigarettes are bad for you. If you are a smoker, you've probably tried to stop, possibly more than once. It's not an easy endeavor, but now you have special motivation to quit and make it stick. In addition to the health risks smoking exposes you to, such as cardiovascular disease, lung cancer, and high blood pressure, it can also have dire consequences for your baby.

According to the U.S. Surgeon General, women who smoke place their child at increased risk for premature birth and stillbirth as well as prenatal complications such as premature rupture of membranes (PROM), placenta previa, placental abruption, and intrauterine growth retardation (IUGR) (for more on prenatal complications, see Chapter 13). The dangers continue after birth, with an increased risk of sudden infant death syndrome (SIDS), low birth weight, recurrent ear infections, and of later development of psychosocial problems such as conduct disorder and substance abuse. Even environmental exposure to tobacco smoke can be detrimental; secondhand smoke causes a slightly increased risk of both IUGR and low birth weight. Cigarettes take a toll on the pocketbook as well; neonatal costs attributable to smoking accounted for $367 million in 1996, tacking an estimated $700 onto the medical costs of the offspring of smoking mothers.

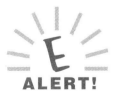

ALERT!

Studies have shown that women metabolize nicotine faster in pregnancy, meaning that you may actually require a larger dose of nicotine replacement therapy (NRT) than you would if you weren't pregnant. For this reason, your doctor should oversee the use of any NRT product to ensure its efficacy.

If you're a smoker, ideally you will kick the habit in the planning stages of your pregnancy. However, the good news is that even if you're pregnant and still smoking, quitting now can make a big difference to your baby's health. Women who stop smoking in the first trimester of pregnancy greatly reduce the risk of IUGR for their child. For women who have difficulty quitting through education programs and other conventional means, nicotine replacement therapies—such as gum, patches, or inhalers—may be an option. Although these products are now available without a prescription, be sure to ask your doctor if you are considering their use. You should know that the safety and effectiveness of NRT in pregnancy has not been extensively tested, and animal studies have indicated that nicotine exposure in the womb may cause later breathing problems in offspring. However, for the mother-to-be who smokes heavily and is not able to stop through traditional cessation programs, their use is preferable to cigarettes since they do not contain carbon monoxide or any of the other hundreds of toxic chemicals contained in cigarette smoke.

Avoiding Alcohol

So what about alcohol? You may have heard that a drink or two a week is safe in pregnancy, as long as your consumption is moderate. The truth is that *there is absolutely no known safe level of alcohol intake in pregnancy*, and even a single beer or glass of wine may have an impact on the development of your unborn child. Bottom line—complete abstinence is the safest route for baby. That said, if you have had a cocktail since conception, perhaps before you even discovered you were pregnant, there is no point in obsessing over it. Letting the incident consume you with guilt or allowing it to become a source of undue stress is bad for you and baby. Focus your energies on living a healthy lifestyle now instead.

The consequences of continued alcohol use or abuse during pregnancy include miscarriage, birth defects, developmental problems, and fetal alcohol syndrome (FAS). Babies born with FAS experience growth retardation and central nervous system problems, and develop characteristic facial features, including small eye openings, a small head, a short upturned nose, absence of the groove between the upper lip and the nose, and an undeveloped outer ear. FAS is permanent and irreversible.

Central nervous system (CNS) involvement can cause tremulousness, an inability to suck in newborns, hyperactivity, low IQ, behavioral problems, learning disabilities, and language delays. Alcohol consumption in the first trimester of pregnancy is responsible for the facial anomalies of FAS, while growth retardation and CNS problems can be triggered by drinking at any point in pregnancy. Children who only have some of these symptoms (e.g., CNS problems and growth retardation, but not facial anomalies) may be classified as having fetal alcohol effects (FAE), alcohol-related neurodevelopmental disabilities (ARND), or alcohol-related developmental disabilities (ARDD). The U.S. Centers for Disease Control (CDC) estimates that an average of one in every 1,000 live births results in FAS at a cost of almost $2 billion annually.

Since the first 8 weeks of pregnancy are a time of rapid development for the limbs, heart, central nervous system, and other organ systems of the embryo, it's important to get a handle on binge or frequent drinking (the drinking patterns thought to have the most detrimental effect on your developing baby) now before it's too late. Talk to your health care provider about treatment options, or turn to your church or local social service agency for support.

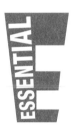

If you have a drinking or substance abuse problem, seeking help early in your pregnancy is imperative. Alcoholics Anonymous can be a source of steadfast support and inspiration. It also has the added benefit of being free of charge and easily accessible, with over 50,000 groups in the United States. Your local chapter can connect you with a meeting in your area, or call the North American A.A. General Service Office at ☎ 212-870-3400.

Eating Right

In pregnancy, women require an extra 300 calories above their normal daily intake to meet the needs of their growing baby. The quality of those calories is particularly important; your developing child requires an extra boost of a variety of vitamins and minerals (see the Recommended Daily Allowance, or RDA, chart below). Most of these nutrients are best served up in your regular diet. Start making it a habit to check nutrition labels in the grocery store, and invest in a good pocket-sized nutrition guide to help you choose produce and other nonlabeled items. However, you will probably require a supplement to meet your iron needs, which double in pregnancy (to 30 mg/daily).

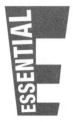

You may find yourself snacking more in pregnancy, either to keep morning sickness at bay or because your growing baby is leaving less and less room for a full stomach. Smaller, more frequent mini-meals can also help combat indigestion and heartburn. Try snacks with a protein punch such as peanut butter on whole-wheat crackers or yogurt with wheat germ swirled in.

Iron helps manufacture an adequate supply of hemoglobin, important for pregnant moms, who experience a 40 to 50 percent increase in blood volume during pregnancy. Your unborn baby is also storing iron that will last for the first few months of life outside your womb. Baby takes what it needs first from your store of iron, so she won't suffer if your intake is inadequate. However, you will end up with anemia, a red blood cell deficiency that can make you feel tired and makes it harder for your blood to carry oxygen throughout your body and to the baby. To combat anemia, eat a variety of iron-rich foods like liver, red meat, fish, poultry, enriched breads and cereals, green leafy vegetables, eggs, and dried fruits. Your health care provider will recommend an iron-enriched prenatal vitamin or iron supplement to make up the difference.

Take iron supplements between meals with plenty of water to eliminate some of the common side effects of constipation, diarrhea, and nausea. If constipation is a problem, add prune juice or other high fiber sources to your diet. To enhance absorption of iron, take your supplement with a fruit juice rich in ascorbic acid (vitamin C), such as orange juice. Remember that tea and coffee contain substances that can inhibit your absorption of iron (as well as calcium), so try to avoid using these to wash down supplements or as an accompaniment to iron-rich foods.

Another critical nutrient in pregnancy is folic acid (folate), which significantly lowers your baby's risk of developing neural tube defects (birth defects of the brain and spinal cord, such as spinal bifida and anencephaly). Because the neural tube forms during the first 4 weeks of pregnancy before many women even realize they are pregnant, the CDC recommends that *all* women of childbearing age get at least 400 micrograms (mcg) of folic acid daily. Pregnant women, and women planning a pregnancy, in particular should get 400 micrograms daily of folic acid in food or supplement form.

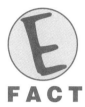

FACT

Each year approximately 2,500 babies are born with neural tube defects. Up to 70 percent of these defects could be prevented by adequate intake of folic acid, yet according to a 2001 March of Dimes survey, only 29 percent of American women of childbearing age take a daily multivitamin containing folate to ensure that they meet the daily requirements.

Foods rich in folate include orange juice, enriched breads and grain products, leafy green vegetables, and dried beans. Since 1998, the U.S. Food and Drug Administration (FDA) has required that grain products such as enriched breads, pastas, rice, and corn meal also be fortified with this important nutrient. Today, there are dozens of breakfast cereals on the market that contain 100 percent of the daily value of folic acid, and just one bowl each morning could make a big difference to your baby's health. Most prenatal vitamins include the RDA of folic acid, as well.

Women's Recommended Daily Allowance (by age)				
	15–18	19–24	25–50	51+	In Pregnancy
Calories	2200	2200	2200	1900	+300
Calcium	1200mg	1200mg	800mg	800mg	1200–1500mg
Folate	180mcg	180mcg	180mcg	180mcg	400mcg
Iron	15mg	15mg	15mg	10mg	30mg
Protein	44g	46g	50g	50g	60g
Riboflavin	1.3mg	1.3mg	1.3mg	1.2mg	1.6mg

Women's Recommended Daily Allowance (by age) *(cont'd)*				
	15–18	19–24	25–50	51+	In Pregnancy
Selenium	50mcg	55mcg	55mcg	55mcg	65mcg
Thiamin	1.1mg	1.1mg	1.1mg	1.0mg	1.5mg
Niacin	15mcg	15mcg	15mcg	13mcg	17mcg
Vitamin B_6	1.5mg	1.6mg	1.6mg	1.6mg	2.2mg
Vitamin B_{12}	2.0mcg	2.0mcg	2.0mcg	2.0mcg	2.2mcg
Vitamin C	60mg	60mg	60mg	60mg	70mg
Vitamin E	8mg	8mg	8mg	8mg	10mg
Vitamin K	55mcg	60mcg	65mcg	65mcg	65mcg
Zinc	12mg	12mg	12mg	12mg	15mg

RDAs from the Office of Women's Health of the U.S. Department of Health and Human Services

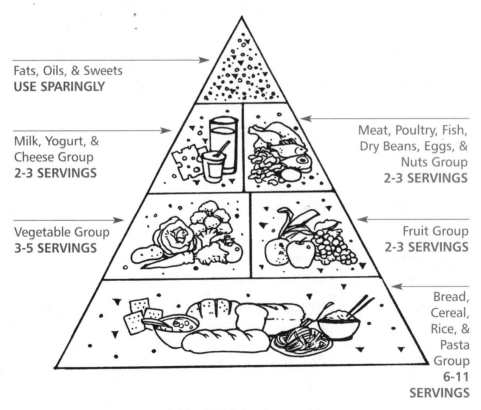

Fats, Oils, & Sweets
USE SPARINGLY

Milk, Yogurt, & Cheese Group
2-3 SERVINGS

Meat, Poultry, Fish, Dry Beans, Eggs, & Nuts Group
2-3 SERVINGS

Vegetable Group
3-5 SERVINGS

Fruit Group
2-3 SERVINGS

Bread, Cereal, Rice, & Pasta Group
6-11 SERVINGS

▲ The USDA food pyramid.

If you aren't a numbers person, or feel overwhelmed by the thought of logging every item that passes your lips, don't worry. Take your prenatal supplement as prescribed by your doctor to bank those vitamins and minerals, then follow a few simple guidelines to ensure that you and baby get your daily fuel. First, ask your health care provider for a copy of the United States Department of Agriculture (USDA) food pyramid chart, and keep it on your refrigerator, in your bag, or anywhere else where it will be easily accessible when you make meal choices. Then, use the pyramid serving suggestions as a minimum guide for a balanced, healthy diet. Be sure to touch base with your provider about how your individual nutrition needs may vary if you have a food allergy or other health condition requiring a special diet.

Exercising Your Body

Women who work out regularly or participate in sports are often worried about whether or not they can continue their routine with a baby on board. In most cases, exercise is not only allowed, it's encouraged. Revised exercise guidelines issued by the ACOG in January 2002 recommend 30 minutes of moderate exercise activity daily for women who are pregnant (excluding high-risk pregnancies). All pregnant women, especially those in high-risk pregnancies and those who were inactive prior to pregnancy, should speak with their physician about exercise options.

Vigorous team sports that pose a risk of injury to you or baby should be avoided (e.g., basketball or soccer). Scuba diving is also not advised because of the risk of decompression sickness. However, swimming, walking, and cycling are ideal ways to stay fit throughout pregnancy. Your local YMCA or community health center may also offer special exercise programs geared toward the prenatal set.

Always stay well hydrated when you work out, and try to confine exercise to the coolest parts of the day in the summer months. An excessive rise in core body temperature (hyperthermia), particularly in the first trimester, has been associated with birth defects. If you feel yourself getting warmer than is comfortable, stop your exercise routine and cool down.

Using Medications and Supplements

Medication use in pregnancy is a thorny issue. There is simply not enough long-term clinical data available on most drugs to provide a 100 percent guarantee of their safety. Ideally, you should avoid all prescription and over-the-counter drugs, except for your prenatal supplements, throughout pregnancy. However, that's an unrealistic expectation given a U.S. Food and Drug Administration (FDA) study that found that women over age 35 take an average of five prescription drugs in pregnancy (the average for women under 35 is three). And if you have a chronic disease, such as diabetes, schizophrenia, or HIV, you have little choice but to continue your treatment, although some modifications may be made by your doctor to minimize the risk to your baby.

The FDA has a classification system for drugs based on the degree of known risk a medication presents to a fetus, but it provides limited information. Acknowledging the need for a more useful ratings system, the agency appointed a Pregnancy Labeling Task Force in 1997 to explore improvements to pregnancy-related drug labeling, a program that was still in development as of the writing of this book. The following chart outlines the five categories currently used for establishing drug safety in pregnancy.

Category	Description
A	Adequate, well-controlled studies in pregnant women have not shown an increased risk of fetal abnormalities.
B	Animal studies have revealed no evidence of harm to the fetus; however, there are no adequate and well-controlled studies in pregnant women. **OR:** Animal studies have shown an adverse effect, but adequate and well-controlled studies in pregnant women have failed to demonstrate a risk to the fetus.
C	Animal studies have shown an adverse effect and there are no adequate and well-controlled studies in pregnant women. **OR:** No animal studies have been conducted and there are no adequate and well-controlled studies in pregnant women.

Category	Description
D	Studies—adequate, well-controlled, or observational—in pregnant women have demonstrated a risk to the fetus. However, the benefits of therapy may outweigh the potential risk.
X	Studies—adequate, well-controlled, or observational—in animals or pregnant women have demonstrated positive evidence of fetal abnormalities. The use of the product is contraindicated in women who are or may become pregnant.

The consequences of not taking a medication must also be taken into consideration when evaluating the use of a drug. Do the benefits of the drug outweigh the risks to the mother and/or fetus? Can a safer medication be substituted temporarily? Or can the drug be temporarily stopped during the period of time it is known to potentially harm the fetus? With close observation, well-researched prescribing, and careful dosing, the use of medication can proceed safely in many cases.

There are a number of drugs that are teratogens—meaning they have been shown to cause birth defects or other developmental problems in pregnancy. Following is a partial list of some well-known offenders. This list is not all-inclusive and you should discuss all medication use with your practitioner.

- Angiotension converting enzyme inhibitors (ACE inhibitors; prescribed for high blood pressure)
- Accutane (isotreinoin; prescribed for cystic acne)
- Androgens (testosterone, danazol; prescribed for endometriosis)
- Anticonvulsants (prescribed for seizure disorders or irregular heartbeats)
- Atypical antipsychotics (prescribed for schizophrenia and bipolar disorder; linked to risk of neural tube defects)
- Certain antibiotics (including streptomycin and tetracycline)
- Certain anticoagulants (warfarin; to prevent blood clotting)
- Tapazole (methimazole; an antithyroid drug prescribed for hyperthyroidism)

- Aspirin and nonsteroidal anti-inflammatory drugs (NSAIDS; for pain relief) during the last trimester
- Chemotherapeutic drugs (used to treat cancer and skin diseases)
- Diethylstilbestrol (DES; not prescribed for pregnant women since FDA issued a warning in 1971)
- Lithium (used for treatment of depression and bipolar disorder)
- Thalidomide (prescribed for leprosy and inflammatory conditions; in limited use due to its high potential for causing birth defects)

Sometimes women decide to self-treat colds and other illnesses with dietary supplements and herbal and botanical remedies in pregnancy, mistakenly assuming that medicine from a botanical source is inherently safe for their fetus. Remember: "Natural" doesn't necessarily mean harmless; herbs can be potent medicinal substances. Even seemingly benign substances like herbal tea have the potential to interact with other foods and medications and cause harm to your developing child. Always check with your care provider before taking anything medicinal, herbal, or otherwise.

On Your Mind

Although physical wellness and mental health are often perceived as two separate and distinct things, the truth is that the mind and body are inextricably linked and what impacts one usually affects the other as well. This connection is particularly strong in pregnancy as the rapid physical changes taking place alter the biochemical balance of the body and brain. Pregnancy is also a precursor to one of the biggest life-changing events there is—the arrival of a baby—and that alone is enough to stir up new and unexpected feelings.

Emotional Health

The hormonal changes that occur in pregnancy can have you feeling weepy one minute and irritable the next. And the emotions you experience, especially the negative ones, can be detrimental to your growing child. Depression, stress, and anxiety may alter your eating and sleep patterns, robbing you and baby of the nutrients and rest you need.

Clinical studies have found that depression and stress also have a direct impact on fetal growth and infant development. If you are feeling blue, you aren't alone; up to 10 percent of women experience ongoing antepartum depression and 70 percent have had depressive symptoms at some point in their pregnancy. Yet women frequently feel guilty that they are feeling so bad during a period of their life that is supposed to be joyful, and for that reason many do not seek professional help.

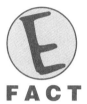

FACT

If you're feeling hopeless, sad, tired, having trouble sleeping, or losing interest in things that used to give you pleasure, you may be experiencing antepartum depression. Research has linked depression during pregnancy to preterm delivery, lower birth weight, developmental problems in infancy, and a 50 percent chance of developing postpartum depression after the baby is born. Don't wait—talk to your provider about treatment options today.

Keeping Stress in Check

Pregnancy is a stressful time. A lot of it is positive, exciting stress as you plan for the baby. But you may also be feeling the pressures of impending financial and family responsibilities, fears of labor and delivery, and new career challenges. Trying to keep up with a hectic prepregnancy schedule as your body grows to a very large and unwieldy size is also a sure-fire way to stress out. In high enough amounts, the stress hormone cortisol can cross the placental barrier and impact fetal brain development. It has also been linked to the development of high blood pressure in animal offspring studies. That's why it's essential to take time out for yourself throughout your pregnancy to decompress (see Chapter 4 for more on stress management).

Genetic Counseling

If you have a history of genetic disease or birth defects in your family or are considered at risk for passing along a hereditary disorder based on your ethnic or racial background, your provider may refer you to a genetic counselor, another tool in the prenatal diagnostic arsenal. Genetic counselors certified by the American Board of Genetic Counseling have a CGC designation after their name, which indicates that they have passed a certification exam, have a graduate degree in genetic counseling, and have logged significant clinical training experience.

What It Is

A genetic counselor takes a detailed family and social history and creates a statistical analysis of your child's risk for acquiring genetic or birth defects. She will also provide you with information on the conditions in question and the risks and benefits of further testing, and will answer any questions you may have. Some of these tests may involve checking you or your partner for carrier genes, while others test the fetus (for more on diagnostic and screening tests see Chapter 5).

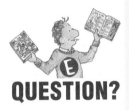

QUESTION?

I'm 40 and pregnant with my second child. What are my chances of an uncomplicated pregnancy?
Women over age 35 have a higher risk for developing diabetes, high blood pressure, and placental problems in pregnancy. There is also an increased risk of having a baby with a chromosomal disorder such as Down syndrome—at age 40 your chances are 1 in 100. The good news is that proper prenatal care can greatly reduce your risk of many birth defects and complications.

What It Isn't

Some women refuse genetic counseling on the grounds that they would never elect to terminate their pregnancy. However, genetic counseling isn't designed to be a "survival of the fittest" venture, but rather a way to help you and your spouse or partner reach an informed decision. A genetic counselor is trained to remain objective and not to attempt to influence your choices. Many couples can and do continue a pregnancy even after testing indicates their child will be born with a serious medical condition or birth defect. Advance knowledge allows a family to prepare emotionally, and to create a suitable environment for a special-needs newborn. It can also mean a better outcome for the child to have a medical support network already in place.

For more on genetic tests and screening, see Chapter 13.

Chronic Health Conditions

If you have a chronic health problem such as diabetes, asthma, or heart disease, you will face some special challenges over the next 9 months as your body adjusts to the major remodeling going on inside right now. Remember that your baby's health depends on your well-being, so staying on top of your treatment is essential. It's important to bring your primary health care provider into the pregnancy picture as soon as possible (ideally, when you start planning your pregnancy).

Your doctor may adjust your medication or treatment regimen, and in most cases will want to follow your progress closely. You may also be referred to a perinatologist—an ob-gyn that specializes in high-risk pregnancies. See Chapter 13 for more on chronic illness and high-risk pregnancies.

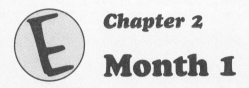

Chapter 2

Month 1

During the first trimester of pregnancy, which lasts approximately 14 weeks from the first day of your last menstrual period, your body is hard at work forming one of the most intricate and complex works of nature. By the end of your first official month of pregnancy (6 weeks after your last menstrual period, but 4 weeks since conception), your developing child will have grown an astonishing 10,000 times in size since fertilization.

Baby This Month

Making its longest journey until the big move 9 months from now, your developing baby (called a zygote, or fertilized ovum) travels from the fallopian tube and into the uterus (or womb). After fertilization, the zygote begins a process of rapid cell division, and by day 4 it has formed a small solid cluster of cells known as a morula (after *moris,* which is Latin for "mulberry"). The morula finishes the trip down the fallopian tube, reaching the uterus about 3 to 4 days after fertilization.

The Blastocyst

By day 5 or 6, your baby takes on its third name change in less than 1 week as the morula grows to a blastocyst. The blastocyst contains two distinct cell layers with a cavity at the center. The inner layer will evolve into the embryo, and the outer layer will develop into the placental membranes—the amnion and the chorion. Within days, the blastocyst nestles into the nutrient-rich lining of your uterus (the endometrium) as implantation begins about 1 week after conception. Wispy fingers of tissue from the chorion layer called chorionic villi will anchor the blastocyst firmly to your uterine wall where they will begin to build a network of blood vessels. These villi are the start of the placenta, a spongy oval-shaped structure that will "feed" the fetus (via the umbilical cord) with maternal nutrients and oxygen throughout pregnancy.

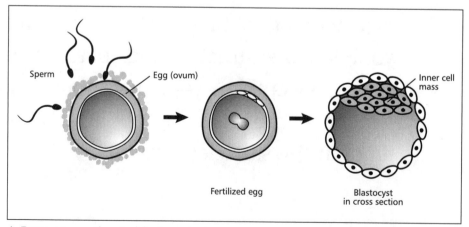

▲ From conception to blastocyst.

The Embryo

About 15 days after conception, the blastocyst officially becomes an embryo. Next to the embryo floats the yolk sac, a cluster of blood vessels that provide blood for the embryo at this early stage until the placenta takes over. The embryo is surrounded by a water-tight sac called the amnion (or amniotic sac). The amniotic fluid that fills the sac provides a warm and weightless environment for your developing baby. It also serves as a sort of embryo airbag (or in this case, fluid bag), protecting baby from the bumps and bustle of your daily routine. Nature efficiently double bags your baby, surrounding the embryo and the amnion with a second membrane called the chorion.

During this first 4 weeks of development, your embryo has laid the groundwork for most of its major organ systems. As month 1 draws to a close, baby's heart is beating (although you won't be able to hear it for several weeks yet), lung buds have appeared, and construction of the gastrointestinal system and liver are well underway. The neural tube, the basis of the baby's central nervous system, has developed and the fore-brain, midbrain, and hindbrain are defined. He (or she) is starting to look more like a person, too. The first layer of skin has appeared, facial features are surfacing, and arm and leg buds—complete with the beginnings of both feet and hands—are visible. It's an amazing list of accomplishments considering your baby is about the size of a raisin (less than ¼ inch long).

Your Body This Month

From your tired and anxious mind to your busy bladder, all of your body's systems may seem to be in overdrive during these early days of pregnancy. The first thing you will notice is the absence of your monthly menstrual period—in many cases, this is what tipped you off to your pregnancy in the first place. Your embryo is secreting the human chorionic gonadotropin (hCG) hormone into your system. In addition to interrupting menstruation, hCG signals the ovaries to produce the hormone progesterone until the eighth week of pregnancy when the placenta takes over production.

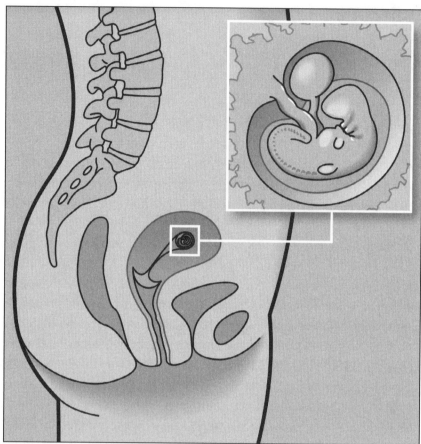

▲ Now an embryo, your baby at month 1 of gestation.

Your Body Changes

At this point in your pregnancy, you might not notice any significant changes in shape and size. Although you aren't menstruating, you feel slightly bloated and your waistband may begin to feel a bit snug. Your breasts may also start to increase in size, and the areolas around your nipples may enlarge and darken. No period? Bigger breasts? This baby is doing wonders for you already! Now for the cloud around that silver lining—fuller breasts are often more tender in pregnancy (although a supportive sports bra can help).

You may also experience increased vaginal secretions similar to those you get premenstrually, another hormonal side effect. These typically last throughout pregnancy and may actually worsen in the third trimester, so stock up on panty liners now. Normal vaginal secretions in pregnancy are clear to white in color, mucus-like, and both odor and pain free. If you experience discharge that is thick, foul-smelling, off-color, or accompanied by itching, blood, or pain, contact your health care provider immediately to rule out infection or other problems.

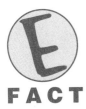

FACT

Some women experience minor vaginal blood flow, called spotting, as the embryo implants itself into the uterine wall. Because of the timing—7 to 10 days after ovulation—it is often mistaken for the beginning of the menstrual period. The spotting, which usually lasts only 1 or 2 days, is pink to brown and may be accompanied by minor cramps.

What You Feel Like

Building a baby is hard work, and even though it's early in the process, it isn't unusual to feel tired and run down right now. If at all possible, try to grab a nap during the day. If that isn't feasible due to a full-time job or other young children at home, make an early bedtime a priority. Although it may run contrary to your nature to be sleeping away the daylight hours when you could be accomplishing one of the 75 other things on your to-do list, thinking of it as a naptime for baby may help. Once you've started down the long road of sleepless nights that new motherhood brings, you'll be longing for the days of early bedtimes and frequent naps!

You may also find yourself spending more and more time in the bathroom. You are urinating more frequently due to high levels of progesterone, which relax your bladder muscles. Unfortunately, frequent urination is one symptom that will likely remain with you throughout pregnancy as your baby grows and the uterus exerts more and more pressure on your bladder. Constipation may become a problem due to increased levels of progesterone; you also may experience problems if you're taking iron supplements (for more on easing constipation, see Chapter 6).

Your cardiovascular system is undergoing big changes right now as it adjusts to meet baby's growing demand for the oxygen and nutrients your blood is carrying. Circulating pregnancy hormones dilate, or expand your blood vessels to accommodate an eventual 50 percent increase in blood volume. Your cardiac output, a measurement of how hard your heart is working to pump blood, increases by 30 to 50 percent, while your blood pressure drops. This is why you may find yourself feeling faint. If you are dizzy or lightheaded, sit or lay down on your side as soon as possible. Try not to lay flat on your back, particularly later in pregnancy as the pressure your uterus places on both the aorta and the inferior vena cava (two of the large blood vessels that help keep oxygen circulating to you and baby) will actually make the dizziness worse.

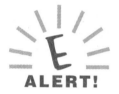

ALERT!

If episodes of fainting or dizziness persist, or are accompanied by abdominal pain or bleeding, contact your health care provider immediately. They could be symptoms of ectopic (or tubal) pregnancy, a potentially fatal condition where implantation occurs outside of the endometrial lining of the uterus (e.g., in the fallopian tubes). See Chapter 13 for more on ectopic pregnancy.

And then, there's the most notorious of all pregnancy symptoms—morning sickness. Referred to by clinicians as nausea and vomiting of pregnancy, or NVP, up to 80 percent of women experience one or both of these symptoms at some point in their pregnancy. As you may know all too well by now, the more accurate term is morning, noon, and night sickness; NVP can happen at any time and strikes with varying intensity. Many women find that their stomach starts to settle as the first trimester draws to a close (anywhere from week 12 to 16), but for others the queasiness persists throughout the entire pregnancy. NVP and relief strategies are covered in depth later in this chapter.

At the Doctor

Set up your first prenatal care visit as soon as you know you are pregnant. For now through the seventh month, you'll be seeing your provider on a monthly basis (unless you are considered high risk, in which case you may have more frequent appointments). If you're seeing a new doctor or midwife, expect your initial visit to be a bit longer than subsequent checkups since you'll be asked to fill out medical history forms and insurance paperwork. Some providers will send you these materials in advance so you can complete them at home. If you still haven't chosen a provider, now is the time to do so.

Your provider will ask plenty of questions about your health history and the pregnancy symptoms you have been experiencing. Make sure that you take advantage of this initial appointment to ask about issues that are on your mind as well. In addition to this interview time, you will undergo a thorough physical examination, give a urine sample (the first of many), and have blood drawn for routine lab work. If you haven't had a Pap smear in the last year, your provider may also take a vaginal swab of cells scraped from your cervix for this purpose. For a detailed look at diagnostic and screening tests in pregnancy, go to Chapter 5.

Your provider will probably supply you with educational brochures and pamphlets on prenatal care, nutrition, office policies, and other important issues. There will be a lot of new information to absorb, so don't feel as though you have to study everything on the spot. However, do take everything home so you can read and refer to it later. Start a folder or notebook for keeping pregnancy information together, and store it near your bed or other favorite reading and relaxation spot for easy access. Add a pad of paper to your "pregnancy portfolio" so you can jot down any questions for your provider.

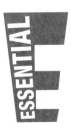

Remember, the dad-to-be is in this pregnancy, too. By all means, bring your spouse or partner to the doctor with you. In addition to providing moral support, he probably has just as many questions about baby as you do. He can also help you remember the things your provider tells you that seem to promptly exit your brain as soon as you leave the examining room.

Confirming Your Pregnancy

Today's home pregnancy tests are highly sensitive (many claim a 99 percent or higher accuracy rate), and provide many women with a convenient and private way to confirm their pregnancy. However, juggling sticks, strips, and tiny plastic cups while trying to decode the magic answer window does leave some room for operator error. If your provider hasn't yet officially confirmed your pregnancy with a lab test, he or she will do so now at this first visit, typically with a urine test, although a blood (or serum) test may be used. The pregnancy test measures the amount of hCG in your system. Urine tests detect levels above 25–50 milli-international units per milliliter (mIU/mL), while the more sensitive serum tests can detect levels as low as 5–10 mIU/mL. Blood tests may be performed in cases where a urine test is negative but pregnancy is still suspected (usually in the early weeks of pregnancy).

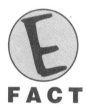

FACT

Because your urine will not start to contain hCG until after the embryo is implanted in the endometrial lining of the uterine wall, a home test will not always detect your pregnancy as early as it may claim. A 2001 study published in the *Journal of the American Medical Association* found that 10 percent of clinical pregnancies were undetectable the first day of a missed menstrual period using a urine hCG test.

Estimating Your Due Date

While pregnancy lasts approximately 280 days, or about 9 calendar months, your estimated date of delivery (or EDD) is based on a 10 "lunar month" pregnancy. Each month is four 7-day weeks. Why lunar months instead of following a good old fashioned calendar? Lunar months are based on a 28-day menstrual cycle, which is considered the average cycle length.

It's important to remember that most providers determine gestational age (how far along you are) from the first day of your last menstrual period (called LMP). This means that you are officially 2 weeks pregnant at the moment of conception. How's that for an existential twist? Of course, if your cycle is longer or shorter than 28 days, or if you have an irregular menstrual period, some mathematic gymnastics are required. In addition, if you're hazy on the date of your LMP, the EDD could be harder to pinpoint. Refer to Appendix C for an estimated due date table.

Because this is all so confusing, your provider probably makes good use of the preprinted EDD charts in her office. However, if you do have a regular 28-day cycle, you can figure out your own EDD by taking the date of your last period, counting 3 months back, and then adding 7 days. For example, if your last period began on September 1, you would go back through August, July, and into June. Then add 7 days to come up with an estimated due date of June 8. An alternate method is to count 280 days (40 weeks) from the first day of your last period.

Prenatal Vitamins

While some experts question whether you need to supplement a well-balanced diet with a vitamin and mineral supplement, most practitioners feel that a daily prenatal vitamin can't hurt, and in many cases will benefit you and your developing fetus. A basic prenatal vitamin contains vitamins A, D, E, C, B_1, B_2, B_6, B_{12}, calcium, copper, iron, magnesium, zinc, and folic acid (other vitamins and minerals may be included). At a minimum, it is recommended that you take a daily dose of 400 micrograms of folic acid to prevent neural tube defects in the first trimester, plus other essential nutrients such as iron and calcium. Some women find prenatal vitamins, which are the rough equivalent of a horse pill, tough to swallow (literally). And if you're experiencing morning sickness, you may find them hard to keep down. Try experimenting with different brands and formulations—there are chewable and flavored versions of prenatal vitamins now on the market. Your provider probably has a roomful of vitamin samples for the asking, so request some freebies if they aren't offered. Taking the vitamins at night may also reduce nausea.

Learning the Ropes

At each appointment, you'll provide a urine sample, have a weigh-in, and get your blood pressure taken. Other diagnostic and screening tests may also be administered throughout pregnancy (for more on these look ahead to Chapter 5). Once you're in the examining room, you may or may not have to disrobe depending on your provider's policy and how far along you are. For your first prenatal visit you will probably don a gown for a full physical exam. Later, some providers will simply have you move your clothing aside for a quick belly check and measure, while others prefer a more thorough examination (e.g., checking your heart rate, examining your feet for any swelling).

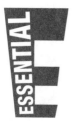

Get to know the support staff in your provider's office. Not only will it make your visits a more pleasant experience, it provides you with an invaluable personal contact when you're trying to squeeze in an unexpected appointment, experiencing insurance difficulties, or having trouble reaching your doctor.

When to Call the Doctor, Day or Night

At your first appointment, your provider may discuss how patient phone calls are handled both during the day and after hours. Frequently, obstetrical practices use a triage system where the receptionist or intake coordinator answers and prioritizes calls and has a nurse, midwife, or physician return them in order of urgency. If your doctor is in the office and you feel more comfortable speaking with him directly (and don't mind waiting a little longer for your answer, if necessary), be sure to make your preferences known when you call.

Usually an answering service will pick up after-hours calls and will page the doctor or midwife on duty who will then return your call. In most group practices, providers usually take turns covering nights and weekends, so you will get a call back from the on-call practitioner. If you aren't given any guidelines for reaching staff after hours, make sure you ask.

Call your doctor immediately if you experience any of the following symptoms:

- Abdominal pain and/or cramping
- Fluid or blood leaking from the vagina
- Abnormal vaginal discharge (e.g., foul-smelling, green, or yellow)

- Painful urination
- Severe headache
- Impaired vision (e.g., spots, blurring)
- Fever over 100.4 degrees Fahrenheit
- Chills
- Excessive swelling of face and/or body
- Severe and unrelenting vomiting and/or diarrhea

You should also become familiar with the signs of preterm labor (covered in Chapter 13). Some women hesitate to pick up the phone for fear that they're being oversensitive or a hypochondriac. While a good dose of common sense should be used in contacting your doctor after hours (for example, a call regarding the pros and cons of epidurals is probably not a good idea at 3 A.M.; unless you're in labor, of course), in most cases "better safe than sorry" applies. Remember, your provider works for you, and you're heading up this pregnancy team. Learn to trust your instincts. If something just doesn't feel right to you, make the call.

On Your Mind

Pregnancy, particularly a first pregnancy, is a time of great anticipation as you head out into uncharted waters. Now that you've been to your first prenatal appointment and have officially started this journey, you may be surprised to find yourself filled with conflicting emotions.

Elation and Excitement

If this is a planned pregnancy, particularly a long-fought and hard-earned one, you may be thrilled beyond belief. Of course, even the little surprises can be sources of great joy. You are creating a new and unique life of boundless potential. As a family, you will share your hopes, dreams, knowledge, and love. This is one of the most important tasks—and special experiences—of your life. So excitement, and even a few high fives, is the order of the day.

If you haven't shared the good news with your other children or family members yet, look ahead to Chapter 11 for some tips.

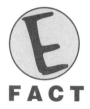

FACT

Feeling drippy? Pregnancy hormones may have you producing excess saliva, a condition called ptyalism. Postnasal drip and/or congestion is another common side-effect of hormonal changes. Both of these may be at least partial contributors to an unsettled stomach, or morning sickness.

Anxiety

Worries about the baby's health, and the possibility of miscarriage, are common fears early in pregnancy. If you've had a previous miscarriage, you may be walking on eggshells trying to second-guess every move you make. The good news is that knowing your history of miscarriage, your provider is following your progress closely.

Although it may be easier said than done, letting go of your anxieties, at least for a little while, is the best thing for you and your baby right now. Try designating a certain area of your home, like your bedroom, a "worry-free" zone, and then stick to a vow to let your anxieties go when you are in that space. Use sounds, sights, and smells to make it as comfortable and relaxing as possible. An aromatherapy candle you like, soft music or nature sounds, and some soothing scenery in the form of photographs and posters can do wonders for your state of mind. (For more on miscarriage and problems in pregnancy, see Chapter 13.)

You may also be concerned about your ability to provide and care for your child. It's important to remember that good parents learn with experience, and by the experiences of others. The very fact that you're reading this book and getting regular prenatal care shows that you want the best for your baby. By the time your little bundle arrives, you'll be surprised at how much you've learned in the relatively short space of 9 months.

Morning Sickness

Your stomach flutters, then lurches. As your mouth starts to water, you run for the bathroom for the fifth time today. Sound familiar? Morning sickness—called nausea and vomiting of pregnancy (NVP) by the medical profession—is arguably the most debilitating and prevalent of pregnancy symptoms. While most women find that NVP symptoms subside or stop as the first trimester ends, for some they continue into the second and even third trimester. If you're having twins or more, your NVP may also be longer and more intense.

The exact cause of NVP has not been pinpointed, but theories abound. Some possible culprits: the human chorionic gonadotropin (hCG) hormone that surges through your system and peaks in early pregnancy; a deficiency of vitamin B and B_6; hormonal changes that relax your gastrointestinal tract and slow digestion; and immune system changes. Another hypothesis is that morning sickness is actually a defense mechanism that protects both mother and child from toxins and potentially harmful microorganisms in food. No matter what the trigger, it's a miserable time for all.

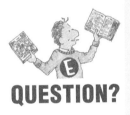

QUESTION?

I can't stand wearing what was my favorite perfume anymore! Can pregnancy cause your nose to go haywire? Pregnancy causes a heightened sensitivity to certain odors—coffee, cigarette smoke, and fried foods are frequent offenders—that can contribute to stomach unrest. One theory is that these olfactory aversions are your body's way of keeping you away from substances that could harm your developing baby.

Remedies and Safety

The following treatments have been associated with some success in lessening symptoms of NVP in clinical trials. (Speak with your health care provider before adding any new supplements to your diet.)

- Ginger. Ginger snaps and other foods and teas that contain ginger (*Zingiber officinale*) may be helpful in settling your stomach.
- Acupressure wristbands (Sea-Bands). Sometimes used to ward off motion and sea-sickness, these wristbands place pressure on what is called the P6, or Nei-Kuan, acupressure point. Available at most drugstores, they are an inexpensive and noninvasive way to treat NVP.
- Vitamin B and B_6. Thiamine (B_1) and B_6. These supplements have

reduced NVP symptoms in several clinical trials. It has been suggested that NVP is a sign of B vitamin deficiency.

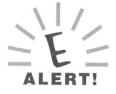

ALERT!

Kava-Kava (*Piper methysticum*), licorice root (*Glycyrrhiza glabra*), rue (*Ruta graveolens*), Chinese cinnamon (*Cinnamomum aromaticum*), and safflower (*Carthamus tinctorius,* or saffron) are just a few of the many botanical remedies that are known to be dangerous in pregnancy. Don't pick up that supplement or cup of herbal tea without asking your health care provider first.

Other treatments that women report as helpful include:

- **Eating smaller, more frequent meals.** An empty stomach produces acid that can make you feel worse. Low blood sugar causes nausea as well.
- **Choosing proteins and complex carbohydrates.** Protein-rich foods (e.g., yogurt, beans) and complex carbs (e.g., baked potato, whole grain breads) are good for the two of you and may calm your stomach.
- **Eat what you like.** Most pregnant women have at least one food aversion. If broccoli turns your tummy, don't force it. The better foods look and taste, the more likely they are to stay down.
- **Drink plenty of fluids.** Don't get dehydrated. If you're vomiting, you need to replace those lost fluids. Some women report better tolerance of beverages if they are taken between meals rather than with them. Turned off by water and juice right now? Try juicy fruits like watermelon and grapes instead.
- **Brush regularly.** Keeping your mouth fresh can cut down on the excess saliva that plagues some pregnant women. Breath mints may be helpful too.
- **Talk to your provider about switching prenatal vitamins.** If it makes you sick just to look at your vitamin, perhaps a chewable or other formulation will help. Iron is notoriously tough on the stomach, so your provider might also recommend a supplement with a lower or extended release amount. And if you can't keep your vitamin down no matter what you try, your doctor may suggest forgoing it for now until your NVP has passed.

How to Cope

Constant queasiness and vomiting may have you wondering why on earth you got pregnant in the first place. Try to take solace in the fact that for most women, NVP is primarily a first trimester affair. Stick close to home and take it easy if at all possible. When staying home isn't an option, talk to your employer about allowing some flexibility with your work schedule. If your stomach is at its worst first thing in the morning, ask about starting later in the day on a temporary basis. Depending on your occupation, working from home some days may be an option. For more on working through pregnancy, see Chapter 9.

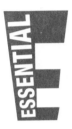

Put together a morning sickness survival kit for the car. Items to include: wet wipes, tissues, small bottle of water; travel-sized toothbrush and toothpaste, a package of gum or breath mints, graham or soda crackers, and a bundle of large freezer-grade zipper lock baggies (for obvious reasons!). For longer trips, a cell phone and a "just-in-case" change of clothes are a necessity.

When It May Be More Than Morning Sickness

When your body can't get the energy it needs from food, it will start to metabolize stored fat. This condition, called ketosis, generates ketones that circulate in your bloodstream and can harm your fetus. Your doctor may test your urine for ketones if you're having severe and persistent nausea and vomiting.

A small percentage of pregnant women (0.3 to 3 percent) experience a severe form of morning sickness called hyperemesis gravidarum (excessive vomiting of pregnancy). If you can't keep any food or fluids down, are losing weight, and are finding it impossible to function normally, you may be in this category. Even though hospitalization is sometimes required for hyperemesis gravidarum, the good news is that the treatment—intravenous fluids to restore fluid and electrolyte balance and in some cases, antiemetics (drugs to stop vomiting)—is relatively simple. If you are prescribed antiemetics, talk with your doctor about the safety data on the drug you are prescribed and any potential effects on the fetus.

Just for Dads

Fathers have their own unique role in pregnancy. While you may not be physically carrying this child (likely a source of enormous relief as you watch your partner struggle with morning sickness and other pregnancy fun), you are sharing the emotional weight of pregnancy, experiencing the same fears, joys, and occasional bewilderment as your significant other. You also have the added responsibility of being her primary source of support in many cases. In fact, this may be the first time in your lives when she is in charge of the manual labor and you're the emotional caregiver. Try to enjoy this new vantage point—think of it as training for life as a dad.

This Wild Ride Called Pregnancy

Although your partner might not look very pregnant yet, chances are she's acting like it. Mood swings, "emotional lability" in medical terms, are the result of the many hormonal changes pregnancy brings and may be one of the first things you notice. So if you're laughing together one minute and being yelled at the next, don't take it personally. It's all part of the package.

Morning sickness, particularly when it is severe, can be a disturbing part of pregnancy for men. Supporting your partner during this difficult time—making sure she gets adequate rest, taking care of household duties, and catering to her food requests, no matter how odd they may seem—is the best way you can help both her and your child.

Fear of the Future

It's natural to feel rattled about providing for an utterly dependent and very tiny person. Practical matters, like being able to support a bigger family, may be dominating your thoughts right now. If you haven't already, talk with your spouse or partner about your concerns; chances are she shares many of the same anxieties as you do and working together as a family is the best way to face them head on. Ⓔ

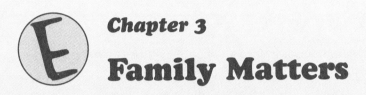

Chapter 3

Family Matters

No matter what shape and size your current household is, a new baby in your home will touch your life in ways you never imagined. Just about every aspect of your daily routine is going to change—how you eat, sleep, play, and work. As you wait to welcome your child to the world, use the time to lay the foundation for your new family circle.

Make Room for Baby

Kids are remarkably adaptable. They can thrive in just about any location, given a healthy and nurturing environment. They do need a safe space to grow in, however; babies in particular learn through exploring and experiencing their surroundings.

A Space of Their Own

Start thinking about where your baby will be sleeping (or not sleeping) and playing so you can coordinate logistics and gear. Keep an open mind, however. Even if you can't wait to see your little angel peacefully dozing against his color-coordinated crib sheets, you may have second thoughts about having him "all the way" down the hall once he arrives (especially when the 2 A.M. feeding rolls around).

Some parents choose to keep their newborn in their room, either in a crib or bassinet or in the parental bed—a somewhat controversial practice known as co-sleeping. Proponents of co-sleeping say that it encourages breastfeeding, boosts milk production, and provides a better bonding experience for parents and baby. Critics cite studies that conclude that bed sharing disrupts sleep patterns and increases the risk of sudden infant death syndrome (SIDS). However, factors such as sleep position, type of bedding, and parental smoking and alcohol consumption raise SIDS risk as well, and it isn't completely clear whether bed sharing in the absence of these risk factors still presents a significant hazard.

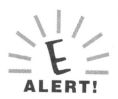
ALERT!

Make sure baby sleeps safe on a firm mattress, without soft bedding or duvets. Always place him on his back to sleep, and never share a bed with a baby after you have been drinking or if you are under the influence of drugs that alter consciousness.

Whatever you decide regarding sleeping arrangements (and you may not decide until you actually have her in your arms), if you have the space you're probably already laying plans for the baby's room. If you're torn about giving up your study for a nursery (after all, she's small—how much space can she need?), think about the baby basics (crib, changing area, dresser) plus all the inevitable *stuff* you're bound to acquire—swings, stuffed animals, bouncy chairs, baby books, bathtubs—and the choice becomes clear.

If a nursery isn't an option due to the size of your home or financial considerations, there are several ways to give baby a place of her own. A folding screen (or two) or curtains hung from a ceiling track can be a creative way to close off part of a room. If you have the money, but limited room, think of building out a wall for a more permanent partition.

Wherever it is, the baby's space should be well ventilated and insulated. Evaluate the area for safety hazards such as peeling paint, dangling blind cords, and loose flooring. If there are doorstoppers installed, make sure they are one-piece; the rubber bumper on many models represents a choking hazard. When it comes time to purchase a crib, make sure that it has no decorative features that could potentially catch on clothing or entrap the baby, and that the crib slats are a maximum of $2^3/8$ inches apart. The mattress should fit snugly against the crib sides.

Bye Bye Miata, Hello Minivan

Time to face the cold hard facts—that sporty two-seater just isn't going to hack it once you have both a baby and all her associated cargo to carry about town.

You don't need to run out and buy a Humvee, but you should cast a critical eye toward your current vehicle and make sure it meets both the practical and safety concerns of your growing family. Some things to look for:

- **Sit back and be safe.** The best place for any child is the back seat. If you have the choice, avoid pickup trucks or other vehicles that don't offer one.
- **Preferred seating.** Size matters, and so does shape. Make sure your car seat fits properly in the vehicle and there is adequate room if you have more than one child to secure. Remember your little one will ride in a rear-facing car seat until he weighs 20 pounds and is a year old.

- **Passenger air bag on/off switch.** If your new baby must ride in the front passenger seat and there is an air bag, there absolutely *must* be a switch that allows you to disengage the air bag on that side. Permission to install a switch can be obtained from the National Highway Traffic Safety Administration (NHTSA). Check with your state motor vehicle bureau for details.

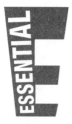

Air bags can save lives, but used improperly they can also cause serious injuries. A rear-facing infant seat places your child's head just inches from the air bag, which deploys with tremendous force and speed—a potentially fatal combination. All kids under 12 should buckle up in the back seat whenever possible.

- **Skip the side air bag.** Side impact air bags can also pose a significant risk of head and neck injury to children. If the vehicle has an activated rear seat side air bag, make sure it has been adequately tested for safe use with children. Otherwise, have it deactivated.
- **Locking seat belts, tethers, or anchors.** Cars built after 1996 should have belts that work with most child seats; always check the owner's manual of any car for child seat belt instructions. Some seats come with locking clips for use with belts in older vehicles. All cars manufactured after September 2002 offer a LATCH system that is independent of the seat belts.
- **Interior trunk release.** If your car was manufactured after September 2001 it should have a release mechanism inside the trunk to prevent curious children from becoming trapped inside. Retrofitted release latches are available for cars without this feature.
- **Don't run hot and cold.** If your heating and cooling system is out of commission, now is the time to get it fixed. You may not mind sweating in summer, but an infant can quickly become overheated. The CDC recommends turning on the car air conditioner in weather 75°F or warmer, and firing up the heater when it dips below 50°F.
- **Accessorize.** Car seat belts and buckles left in the sun can also pose a burn hazard to infants so consider a car seat cover or window and

windshield sun screens, which are also useful in preventing your car interior from absorbing the sun's heat.

Other features that may be helpful but aren't absolutely essential include built-in child car seats and safety door locks.

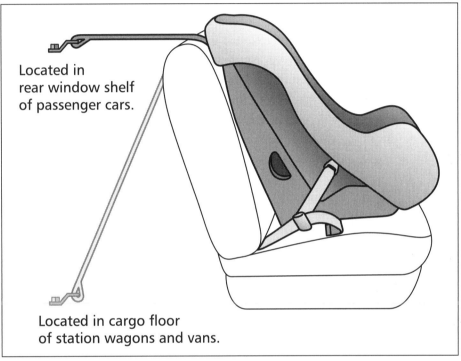

Located in
rear window shelf
of passenger cars.

Located in cargo floor
of station wagons and vans.

▲ The LATCH system—Lower Anchors and Tethers for Children—uses anchors mounted in the seat cushion and a top tether to secure a child safety seat.

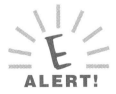

ALERT!

In 93°F weather, a car without air conditioning can reach temperatures in excess of 125°F in just 40 minutes, even with the windows cracked. Because of his small size, a baby's core body temperature rises quickly on a warm day—up to five times faster than that of an adult—and potentially fatal heat-related illness is a serious risk.

Babyproof

Now that you have car safety covered, take a look at potential hazards inside your home.

Although your home safety efforts will undoubtedly pick up steam as your child gets mobile and starts exploring her surroundings, there are some basic things you can do now to protect her in infancy and beyond.

- **Register for recalls.** Take the time to fill out those registration cards for all the baby gear you've received. If a safety recall of the product occurs, the manufacturer will be able to notify you. You can also register for e-mail alerts of new product recalls from the U.S. Consumer Product Safety Commission at *www.cpsc.gov.*
- **Ban cigarettes.** You already know how dangerous it is to smoke during pregnancy, but did you know that secondhand smoke, particularly in a closed home environment, is harmful to your baby's health? Tobacco is also toxic when eaten; since babies put just about everything in their mouths that's just one more good reason to make your home a tobacco-free zone.
- **Get the lead out.** Lead paint, most frequently found in homes built before 1978, is a major hazard to small children. When ingested, either by eating paint chips or breathing lead dust, it can cause CNS damage and a host of other health and developmental problems. Lead solder used in some older plumbing systems can also pose a risk. If you haven't done so already, contact a lead inspector certified by the state and/or the Environmental Protection Agency (EPA) to test your home for the presence of lead and to advise you on abatement procedures, if necessary.
- **Rearrange the furniture.** Block off electrical cords and buy plastic protectors to seal up open outlets. Pad sharp table corners to protect baby from injury. Evaluate your home from a baby's eye view (about three feet off the floor for good measure), and move anything dangerous, expensive, or breakable to higher ground.
- **Practice.** Some old habits—like leaving the toilet seat up—are hard to break. It will be easy to be vigilant later if you get accustomed to baby-safe behavior now. A few new routines to try out: Store

medications, cleaning products, and other toxic substances out of a child's reach; store plastic bags in a latched cabinet; and make sure all members of the household leave the toilet seat (and lid) down.

The High Cost of Having a Baby

If you have substantial or full insurance coverage for your prenatal care and delivery expenses, you can breath a sigh of relief. A 1998 study found that average charges for delivering a baby were $7,090 for an uncomplicated delivery and $11,450 for a cesarean section. Prenatal care adds another several thousand to the bill, but studies show that those expenses are more than offset by improved outcomes for both mother and child.

Insurance Issues

Review your insurance plan so you are clear on the extent and nature of your coverage for both prenatal care and labor and delivery. If you have questions, call your insurance company or speak to the benefits coordinator at your workplace.

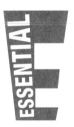

Make sure you find out the procedure for putting the newest member of your family on your health insurance policy once he or she arrives. If you're paying insurance premiums, find out what the additional charge will be so that you can budget for it now.

Keep on top of insurance problems. As any physician's or hospital billing department can tell you, insurance companies do occasionally lose and mishandle claims. Whenever you call either your provider's billing department or the insurance company, take notes summarizing the conversation, including a date to follow up and the name of the person you spoke with. If you're trying to unravel a knotty insurance issue, being able to track it with someone who is familiar with your case will save you time and aggravation. On the other hand, if you aren't getting action, it helps to document exactly who has dropped the ball as you move up the chain of command. Follow up with letters and request written documentation of any actions taken over the phone so you have a paper trail as well.

Payment Options

If you have a large deductible to pay out of pocket, or are responsible for a hefty percentage of your physician's bill, don't panic. Work with your provider's office to negotiate a realistic payment schedule. Contact the business office of the hospital or birthing center you will be delivering at for registration information and details on their billing terms. Some providers and hospitals may have maternity assistance programs, including sliding fee scales and prepayment discounts.

Ways to Save

According to U.S. Census estimates, 14 percent of all Americans were without health insurance in 2000. There are public aid programs available if you are uninsured and unable to meet the financial obligations of prenatal care and childbirth.

Medicaid is a state-run public assistance program that provides medical care to low-income families at little to no cost. For information on qualifying standards, see the federal Centers for Medicare and Medicaid Services Web site at ✍ *http://cms.hhs.gov* or call your state social services department.

The Special Supplemental Nutrition Program for Women, Infants, and Children (WIC) is a federally funded, state-administered program targeted toward nutritionally at-risk women (both pregnant and postpartum) and children up to age 5. WIC provides food vouchers to those who meet qualifying guidelines and have an annual gross household income that does not exceed 185 percent of the federal poverty level (e.g., $33,485 for a family of four in 2002; slightly higher in Alaska and Hawaii).

The State Children's Health Insurance Program (SCHIP) was instituted in 1997 to insure infants and children from families who are financially strained but earn income levels too high to qualify for Medicare. If you're concerned about insurance coverage for your newborn, call ✆ 1-877-KIDS-NOW or visit ✍ *www.insurekidsnow.gov* for more details.

There may be other financial assistance available in your area. Contact your area social services agency for more details.

Bargain Hunters

Even if you've never been one to clip coupons, the expense of keeping baby in diapers and other essentials is a great incentive to start looking for savings. Next time you're at the doctor's office, take a look around the waiting room for product offers. Many "new parent clubs" have cropped up, supported by formula makers, diaper manufacturers, and other baby product companies, and they often recruit members right here at the source.

Some kid-focused retailers also have coupon clubs. Sign up if you'd like to receive free product samples and coupons. One caveat—putting your name on their mailing lists may open you up to a deluge of junk mail from so-called "valued partners." Check out the form you sign for a printed privacy policy if this is a concern; it may offer you an opportunity to opt out of such mailings. Still, some parents find that a heavier mail load is a small price to pay for substantial savings.

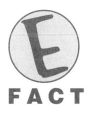

FACT

According to the USDA, 47 percent of infants born in the United States receive nutritional assistance from the WIC program. In 2001, approximately 7.31 million women and children participated in WIC each month. Studies have also shown that WIC participants have better birth outcomes than their peers who did not participate in WIC.

There are several free magazines on the market geared specifically for new parents and moms-to-be, again often available right at your provider's office. Be aware that because these publishers make their money from advertisers rather than subscriptions, they are typically laden with product ads. However, they still have lots of useful new parenting information and an abundance of coupons and freebie offers.

Check your local library for other community or regional parenting publications that can point you toward useful family resources and, again, those handy coupons.

Of course, breast milk is the least expensive way to feed your baby (along with its many other extraordinary health benefits, which are covered in Chapter 19), but if you are planning on bottle-feeding, freebies abound. Formula is expensive, and baby will eventually be putting away about 30 ounces a day, or 900 ounces per month. Acquiring a loyal customer through free samples and other incentives makes good business sense to formula manufacturers, who are big on the aforementioned new parents clubs. They also provide a steady stream of samples to prenatal care providers and pediatricians. If you don't see samples or aren't offered any, ask your provider.

Finally, if you deliver in a hospital, get what you pay for. Chances are you'll be billed for all the items you and your newborn use—including the pacifier, nasal aspirator, sanitary napkins, alcohol swabs, open bags of diapers and wipe cloths, and even the little plastic comb for baby's hair (whether baby has any or not). By all means, take it with you when you leave! Ask the nurse what is fair game. Often the hospital staff can send you home with even more free product samples than you will find in the room.

Financial Planning for a Bigger Family

Hold on to your hats. According to the USDA, a child born in 2001 will cost the average parents between $169,920 to $337,690 by the time he or she reaches age 17 (depending on your income level). If you've been living an unbudgeted lifestyle, now is a good time to start setting up a family spending and savings plan.

Cost Comparisons

Clueless about baby care costs? Do a little detective work and make a reconnaissance mission to the grocery store to gather prices on diapers, wipes, and other essentials. If you're considering day care or an in-home babysitter, now is a good time to get information and monthly cost estimates. As usual, other parents are an excellent source of tips and leads to the best resources in your area.

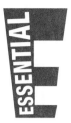

In 1 week, the average baby goes through about 60 to 80 diaper changes. That's a potential pileup of 4,160 diapers in the first year alone! If you're using disposable ones, price cases of diapers at the local warehouse club or discount store since bulk purchases are typically cheaper.

Don't forget to factor pediatric care and additional health insurance premiums into your bottom line. If you belong to an HMO or other managed care health plan, it's probable that well-baby visits are covered at 100 percent or with a minimal co-pay. You may want to review your health insurance options now so that when baby comes you can enroll her in the most appropriate and cost-effective program.

Setting Savings Goals

So now that you've figured out what you'll be spending, what practical use do you put it to? Lay out your current spending habits, including basic monthly bills like utilities and housing, debts that can be downsized (e.g., credit cards and car payments), transportation costs, food and household goods, health care, and discretionary/disposable income. Accounting for everything in black and white will give you a much clearer picture of where you're spending and the size of any gap between income and expenses. It can also help you figure out big-picture questions like whether you have the financial means to switch to a part-time schedule at work.

When it comes time to balance your home budget, be realistic in your planning and prudent when you eliminate discretionary purchases; brown bagging it to work each and every day for the next three years is a noble goal but a weekly or biweekly meal out with colleagues could pay off in other ways. Give yourself a little breathing room for unforeseen emergency expenses like an appliance meltdown or car repairs. A little scrimping here, one less latté a week there, and you'll find budgeting easier than you thought.

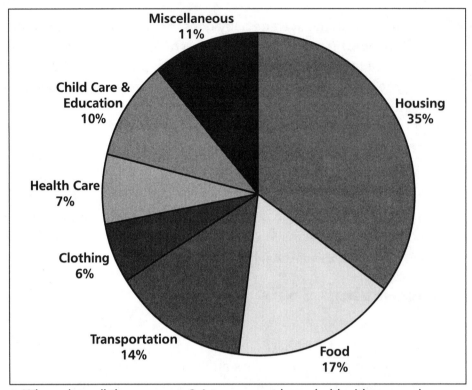

Miscellaneous 11%

Child Care & Education 10%

Health Care 7%

Clothing 6%

Transportation 14%

Housing 35%

Food 17%

▲ Where does all the money go? A two-parent household with a gross income of $52,100 spends an estimated $170,460 to raise a child to age 17.

Some parents find it daunting to consider long-term expenses, like college, when the costs and responsibilities of childrearing itself seem so overwhelming. Just remember that early planning can net big returns over time. According to the U.S. Department of Education, if you start saving just $32 a month in a savings account or other interest-bearing investment at a 4 percent interest rate when your child is born, you will have $10,099 by the time your child is ready to start college. If you don't know an IRA from the NRA, you might want to sit down with a financial advisor to discuss college savings options. He or she may also be able to assist you in re-evaluating your life insurance needs, something else that should be done periodically as your family grows.

Lifestyle Changes, or Stating the Obvious

Your baby's arrival will transform just about everything you think, say, and do. This sea change is probably most evident in first-time parents, who up until now have been enjoying the child-free pursuits of quiet dinners, R-rated movies, and even the occasional wild night out with the girls or boys. Even those moms and dads who are expecting a second or subsequent child will have big adjustments ahead with new challenges like sibling-hood and advanced parental multitasking (e.g., encouraging one child to use his napkin while preventing the other from eating hers). Don't look at it as an end, but rather a new and infinitely more rewarding chapter in your life. You may even find some family pastimes you had never considered before.

Sharing Pregnancy with the Dad-to-Be

With the big focus on mom and her growing belly, it's easy for dads to get overlooked in the pregnancy drama. Remind your significant other that you're in this together. If he isn't quite sure of his role in this new adventure yet, he could be looking to you for cues. Encourage him to join you at prenatal checkups, as well as share pregnancy education and experiences like the first kicks. You should also try to pencil in some special couple time to "talk" to baby, contemplate names, and share your hopes and dreams about your family's future.

From Two to Three

The new person in your life has already started competing for your attention, changing your eating and sleeping patterns and perhaps slowing down your pace. Unexpected emotions may surface between you and your significant other as your pregnancy progresses. He may feel pangs of jealousy at the loss of your "coupledom" and your focus on the baby. On the flip side, you may be feeling as if you're playing second-fiddle to your fetus as he questions the safety of every move you make. Such growing pains are normal. Try to talk about your feelings and approach parenting (even now) as a team effort.

Some dads are intimidated by the size and vulnerability of an infant, and as a result pass most of the child care responsibilities on to the mother, a potential lose-lose situation for both of you. If he is feeling uneasy about his lack of previous experience in the child care arena, suggest a few tag-team babysitting sessions for a niece or nephew or a friend's child to build his confidence.

The Bond of Parenthood

Pregnancy can bring a couple closer together than they ever imagined, but it can also present new frictions in your relationship. The aches and pains of pregnancy would push even the most even-tempered woman to her limits. Add to that a healthy surge of estrogen and progesterone and you have the recipe for major mood swings. Other stressors, like a tepid sex life and financial fears, can also stir the pot. Try to approach these temporary changes with understanding and empathy for your partner, and a healthy sense of humor if at all possible.

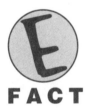

FACT

Strange but true—men can have pregnancy symptoms too. Known as couvade, this sympathy pain phenomenon may have your significant other experiencing nausea, fatigue, weight gain, and mood swings. What's behind it? Anxiety associated with impending fatherhood is suspected by some, but a Canadian study found that men experiencing couvade had distinct hormonal changes that mirrored their pregnant partners.

Single Moms and Support

If you're a single mother-to-be by choice or by circumstance, you aren't alone. About a third of all women (33.2 percent) who gave birth in 2000 were unmarried, according to the U.S. Census Bureau. Pregnancy and birth are physically and emotionally challenging experiences. As a single mom, you may also have the added baggage of financial, career, and custody concerns weighing on you. Dealing with the stress positively is important to you and your baby's health.

Don't fly solo if you don't have to. Enlist a family member or close friend to accompany you on prenatal visits, childbirth classes, and the birth itself. A doula can also be a wonderful source of support for labor and delivery. If at all possible, make arrangements for a live-in companion for the first few postpartum weeks as well.

See Appendix A for more information on support groups for single mothers.

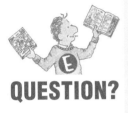

QUESTION?

I'm single, a college student, and pregnant. Where can I turn for financial help?
Some student health insurance programs cover prenatal care and delivery costs, and many schools offer day care facilities that can help you continue your studies once your baby arrives. Check with your university counseling center for more information. You may also qualify for public aid programs like WIC.

An Eye Toward the Future

It may seem worlds away now, but things like school, parks, and playgroups are waiting just around the corner. Don't rush the early years, but as you talk to other parents and families in your neighborhood, start to gather information on the resources available in your area. If you are moving to a bigger home in anticipation of your new arrival, be sure to investigate the school district performance and community resources as part of your house hunting now to save yourself another move in five years.

Kids in Community

That done-to-death proverb, "It takes a whole village to raise a child," is true. The community you raise your child in will play a large part in shaping her values, beliefs, and personality. Of course, you will be the gatekeeper for his early exposures to the outside world, but schools, playgroups, and community services that reinforce your value system will make parenting your older child a group effort rather than a dictatorship. Just as important is your personal investment of time and talents you return to these same institutions.

It's almost never too early to get involved with a playgroup. Your baby will probably enjoy playing with you and observing other kids in a group setting from just a few months old. Investigate what's already available in your area, or talk to some parents and moms-to-be in your neighborhood about starting up something new once baby arrives. Laying the foundation for friendships and positive community relationships now will help your child flourish.

Faith and Family

New parents often find themselves exploring their roots and reconnecting with their own childhood. Even if your family is far away, you can still share the special moments of your pregnancy and birth through photos, videotapes, and phone calls. Sharing the parenting experience across generations can be a powerful experience that forges a special new bond between mother, child, and ultimately—grandchild. And when Thanksgiving comes, you'll finally feel like you belong at the adult table.

When it was just the two of you, spirituality may have taken a back seat in your busy lives. Now that you are going to have a child to raise and educate, the traditions and values of your faith, whatever it may be, are going to take on a new dimension. If you and your partner come from different religious backgrounds, this question holds special significance. Will you choose one organized religion over the other, or expose your child to both faiths? If you're concerned about christening or baptism, an interfaith baptismal service that respects the traditions and beliefs of two-religion families may be an option. The important thing is to open up communications and talk about your expectations now.

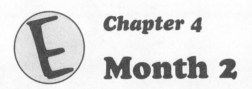

Chapter 4

Month 2

You've made it into month 2, or weeks 6 through 10, of your pregnancy. By the end of this month, your baby will have outgrown its embryonic development and matured into a fetus. Your body is changing rapidly—you may start to feel pregnant now, if you didn't feel so before.

Baby This Month

Your unborn child has now advanced from raisin to raspberry size—about ½ inch in length. By the end of the month, he or she will be about 1 inch long (a good-sized grape). The fetus is lengthening and straightening from the shrimplike, curled form it held last month. The tail she was sporting disappears around week 8, and her closed eyes start to move from the sides of the head to their permanent location. The face is further defined by a nose and jaw, and the buds of 20 tiny baby teeth are present in the gums by week 10. The palate and vocal cords also form around this time, although baby isn't ready to make herself heard just yet.

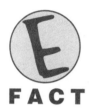

FACT

Boy or girl? Girl or boy? Your child will keep you guessing for at least a few more weeks. While external sex organs begin to differentiate this month, they won't become visible on ultrasound until around week 16 to 20 (and then only with some fetal cooperation). If you're scheduled for an amniocentesis, the gender of your child can be definitively determined at that time. Then again, you may enjoy the element of surprise!

Important organ systems are nearly completed by the end of month 2. The right and left hemispheres of your baby's brain are fully formed and brain cell mass grows rapidly. Soft bones begin to develop, and the liver starts to manufacture red blood cells until the bone marrow can take over the job in the third trimester.

Your unborn baby is also giving his brand new organs a workout. Heart chambers form, the pancreas begins to produce insulin, and the liver secretes bile. The stomach produces gastric juices while the intestines, which have developed in the umbilical cord, move up into the abdomen by the end of the month.

Floating in about 1.5 ounces (approximately 10 teaspoons) of amniotic fluid, your baby has plenty of room for flexing the muscles she is now developing. Because of her small size and spacious accommodations, chances are you won't notice these movements now. At about 18 to 20 weeks, when the second trimester is in full swing and her quarters become a bit closer, you will feel the first flutterings, known as quickening.

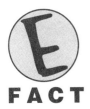

F A C T

If you are at risk for passing on a chromosomal abnormality or hereditary health condition to your child, you may choose to be scheduled for a chorionic villus sampling (CVS) at the end of this month. A CVS is typically administered between weeks 10 and 12, and involves taking a small sample of placental tissue for laboratory analysis. See Chapter 5 for details on CVS procedures and genetic testing.

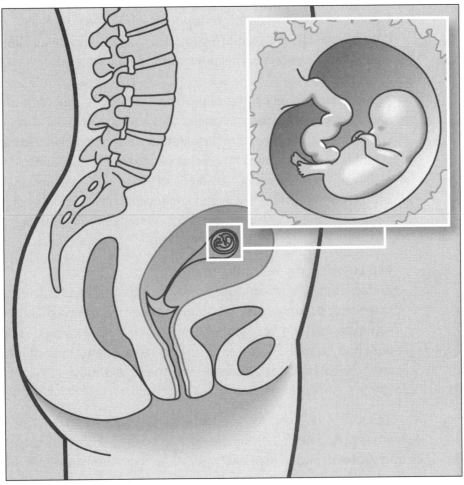

▲ At the end of this month, your baby is officially a fetus.

Your Body This Month

If you weren't feeling very pregnant last month, you are probably starting to now. About midway through this month, hCG levels will begin to peak and then slowly decline as the placenta starts to produce the pregnancy hormones progesterone and estradiol. The ebb and tide of your hormones will trigger a few new pregnancy symptoms this month.

Your Body Changes

Even though you may not have put on any additional weight yet, your growing uterus is pushing the boundaries of your waistline. On average, most women gain between 2.5 to 5 pounds in the first trimester.

Changes in skin and hair are common in pregnancy. Hair that was fine and thin may become thick and shiny during pregnancy, and that fabled pregnancy "glow" may actually be your flawless, blemish-free complexion. On the other end of the spectrum, acne problems and hair breakage and thinning may occur.

Chloasma, also known as melasma, may cause a mask-like darkening or lightening of your facial skin. Freckles and moles are prone to darkening, as well as other pigmented areas of your skin (e.g., areolas). To minimize chloasma and other hyperpigmentation, use a good sunscreen (SPF 30 or higher) to cover exposed skin when you're out in the sun.

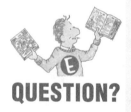

QUESTION?

Will coloring my hair hurt my baby?
To date, there is no conclusive evidence that hair color use in pregnancy is dangerous. If you are concerned over a possible risk, you may opt for a vegetable-based or temporary color treatment until baby is born. Some experts also recommend holding off on all chemical hair treatments during the first trimester.

Your gums may start to bleed when you brush your teeth, a condition known as pregnancy gingivitis. Be sure to floss and brush regularly to keep your teeth and gums healthy. A warm salt-water rinse may soothe swollen gum tissues (ask your doctor first if you have a history of high blood pressure). Now is a good time to schedule a thorough cleaning with your dentist; in a few months, leaning back in a dental chair will be uncomfortable, if not impossible.

What You Feel Like

The stomach rumblings of the first month continue, and an increase in nausea and vomiting may actually occur as hCG levels peak toward the end of this month. On the plus side, your NVP may start to get better in the coming weeks as hCG levels wane. If you're one of those lucky women who do not experience morning sickness at all, you're probably not escaping the feelings of fatigue. Take the hint your body is giving you and take time out to rest.

Other symptoms that may start or continue this month include:

- Frequent urination
- Tender, larger breasts
- Increased vaginal discharge
- Occasional dizziness or faintness
- Indigestion or gas
- Headaches
- Nasal congestion and/or runny nose
- Increased saliva

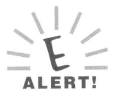

ALERT!

If you have a cat, hand over litter box duties to someone else. Toxoplasmosis, a parasitical infection passed on by infected cat feces and by undercooked meat, has the potential to cause brain damage and other medical problems in your unborn child. Cats also frequent gardens and sandboxes, so wear gloves, and wash your hands thoroughly after working outside.

At the Doctor

If you had your preliminary appointment last month, your prenatal office visits will now start to slip into a routine. At a minimum, expect to step on the scale, give a urine sample, and have your blood pressure checked at the start of each appointment. You'll also be asked about any new or continuing pregnancy symptoms, and your provider will feel the outside of your abdomen to determine the size of your uterus.

Get the Most Out of Monthly Checkups

Bring along that list of questions that have come up since your last visit. Again, write these down when they come to you and your partner so you won't have to rely on your memory in the doctor's office. And make sure your questions are answered before you leave; although it's nice to be asked if you have any concerns, in the busy atmosphere of an obstetrical practice your provider may occasionally forget. Stop her before she leaves the exam room and let her know you have a few questions. Never feel like you're being pushy or overbearing (remember, you're leading this team). In most cases she will do what she can to educate you and reduce any anxieties. If she doesn't, it's never too late to find someone who will.

Tests This Month

Additional blood tests for Rh factor and rubella antibodies may be ordered this month if they were not taken at your last appointment. For more on medical tests in pregnancy, see Chapter 5.

On Your Mind

Now that you're feeling more symptoms of pregnancy, the reality of impending parenthood may suddenly hit home. "So much to do, so little time," you may be thinking. Understanding and recognizing your emotional changes can help you better control your stress levels.

Mood Swings

Find yourself laughing hysterically or sobbing uncontrollably? If you're normally the even-keeled type, these emotional outbursts can be downright alarming. You aren't losing control or losing your mind, you're experiencing the normal mood swings of pregnancy. Although this emotional lability may continue throughout pregnancy, it is typically strongest in the first trimester as you adjust to hormonal and other changes.

Given the transformation your body is going through and the accompanying aches and pains, you have every right to be cranky. In fact, when you factor your physical discomforts with the spectrum of emotions you're experiencing as motherhood approaches, you've got a license to be hell on wheels. Of course, no one is happy when that happens (just ask your partner), so take steps now to reduce your stress level and achieve some balance.

Stress and Stress Management

It's easy to get stressed out over what may seem like an overwhelming amount of preparation for your new family member. Your body is already working overtime on the development of your child; try to keep your commitments and activities at a reasonable level to prevent mental and physical overload.

Controlling outside stress is even more important when your pregnant body is under the physical stress of providing for an unborn baby. And added psychological stress can make the discomforts of pregnancy last longer and feel more severe.

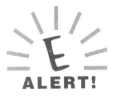

ALERT!

Some traditional stress control methods, such as relaxation techniques involving certain strenuous yoga positions or martial arts, for example, are not appropriate for pregnant women. You should also not try fad diets, herbal preparations, or over-the-counter medications (which are generally not good stress control methods in any case). When in doubt, check with your health care provider.

Anxiety may also impact your child's health. An increase of corticotropin-releasing hormone (CRH), a stress-related substance produced by the brain and the placenta, has been linked to preterm labor and low birth weight. Research has also suggested a possible connection between first-trimester maternal stress and congenital malformations.

As you rush to get everything "just so," remember that your little one is not going to care if the crib matches the dresser, but he will feel the effects of your excess tension. Keeping it all in perspective is important. So is taking steps to decompress when you do feel the pressure building.

Effective stress management involves finding the right technique for *you*. Relaxation and meditation techniques (e.g., progressive muscle relaxation, yoga with your doctor's consent), adjustments to your work or social schedule, or carving out an hour of "me" time each evening to decompress are all ways you can lighten your load. Exercise is also a great stress control method, but be sure to get your doctor's approval regarding the level of exercise that is appropriate for you.

Dressing for Two

Finding maternity clothes that are fashionable, that fit, that grow comfortably with you, and that don't cost a fortune can be a challenge. Start out by deciding how much you want to spend; if you blow your whole clothing budget on a few items, you're going to be awfully limited in your wardrobe.

A few other things to keep in mind while you develop your wardrobe:

- **Consider your laundry threshold.** Check the tags and make sure that the care instructions mesh with your lifestyle. Hand washing your delicates may not top your priority list right now. And make sure you get enough maternity pieces so you aren't washing the same three outfits constantly.
- **Mix and match.** Try to build on what you already own by adding pieces that will work well in a variety of combinations.
- **Keep your sense of style.** Although maternity clothes are getting more fashionable in response to women's needs, there are still plenty of overalls festooned with ruffles and appliqués, "I'm With Fetus" T-shirts, and similar maternity monstrosities out there. Buy what you like; even if it takes a little searching it will be worth it.

- **Built to last?** You'll only be wearing these clothes for a matter of months, so they don't need to be made to withstand a natural disaster. However, if you're planning on stretching their shelf life through another pregnancy, spending a little more on well-made, durable attire is more economical in the long run.

Look Good . . . Feel Good

Dressing well can improve your mood and self-image at a time when it may be shaky. Notice it's dressing *well*, not necessarily dressing up, in whatever your unique style sense calls for. That may mean a favorite jogging suit for running errands or a little (or big) black dress for a night out. Don't forget to purchase some nice loungewear or pajama sets for your take-it-easy days. Even when you're throwing up and miserable, slipping on something cozy can comfort your soul if not your stomach.

Shopping by Due Date

Think about the time of year when you'll be delivering, especially if you live in a region with an inconsistent climate. Being 9 months' pregnant in the dog days of summer wearing the wool pants you bought mid-winter will not be a good thing. To bridge the seasonal shifts, buy clothing that layers—peeled down for summer and piled on for winter. Invest in mix-and-match pieces in breathable fabrics that are adaptable to temperature changes.

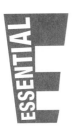

Wondering how you can possibly determine how clothes you buy now will fit you in 6 months? You've never seen a *belly form*, available at most maternity stores. A small pillow that mimics the look of advanced pregnancy, you tie the belly form to your midsection before trying on maternity clothes. An added bonus— you'll get a sneak preview of what you'll be looking like in just a few short months.

Beg, Borrow, and Rent

What could you possibly find in your partner's closet? Plenty, if you use a little imagination. Oversized button-down oxfords and a fashion-forward Hawaiian shirt or two if you're feeling adventurous. Even some of his khakis or other casual slacks may be a good fit in the early months of pregnancy when you're too big for your old pants yet not quite to maternity clothes stage. If you're just starting to show in late summer, but want to save your clothing budget for fall and winter weather attire, borrow a pair or two of his cargo shorts to fill the gap.

If you and your significant other aren't a good size match, tap formerly pregnant friends and family for contributions. Take what you're offered—graciously. Even if it doesn't look quite "you" at the onset, try matching it with some of your own pieces and accessorizing; the diversity may do your meager wardrobe some good.

There is also a new breed of maternity clothing boutique, where for a monthly or weekly fee you can rent a selection of outfits to get you through pregnancy. The biggest benefit—more variety in your wardrobe since you can switch out clothing on a regular basis. The downside—if you're planning on a subsequent pregnancy, you won't have anything to keep and use again for your investment.

Dressed for Success

Women who work in an office or other professional environment have the added challenge and expense of finding clothes for work and play. Because of their limited lifespan in most women's closets, maternity clothes make great resale shop fodder. You may be surprised at some of the bargains you uncover. Consignment stores that deal specifically in maternity wear are also becoming more commonplace; check your local yellow pages to see if there is one near you.

Just for Dads

Things get interesting this month as you both get familiar with the weird but wonderful world of the pregnant body. Step right up and witness the amazing expanding belly. Thrill to the fantastic swelling bustline! Dare to brave the snores and thrashes of the mother-to-be as she tries to find comfort in her natural sleeping habitat. This truly is the greatest show on earth.

Her Changing Body

Getting your libidos in synch during pregnancy can be a challenge. If she's experiencing nausea and vomiting right now, chances are she's not feeling too sexy. On the other hand, for some women the hormonal onslaught of pregnancy has their sexuality in overdrive. You too may feel a similar range of emotions as the pregnancy progresses. Although you may never have thought it possible, fears of somehow hurting the baby during intercourse and a new perception of your partner as a mother may have you shying away from the bedroom. Or, you may find her physical metamorphosis and composure and strength despite it all a highly sensual experience.

So what do you do if you aren't on the same sexual wavelength? First of all, be sympathetic to the physical demands on her body right now, and remember this is a temporary situation. She may be feeling insecure about her appearance, or just awkward and clumsy as her body grows. Stress and anxiety can also douse her sex drive. Reassure her that she's still beautiful, perhaps even more so, and try to lighten her load by pitching in around the house and taking over some of the tasks that may be getting difficult for her (such as bending over to pick up your dirty socks).

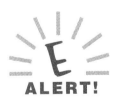

ALERT!

Pregnant women should not have sex if they are having preterm labor, premature cervical dilatation, or complications from a placental previa. Some physicians will tell patients with a twin pregnancy or history of incompetent cervix not to have sex, but these cases are assessed individually based on each woman's circumstances. However, any woman with a pregnancy that is at risk for premature delivery should avoid intercourse.

If she's looking for love, but you aren't, look at the reasons behind your feelings. Is safety a concern? Sex is safe and normal if the pregnancy is progressing normally. The baby is well protected in the uterus. Be aware that an orgasm can sometimes trigger contractions, but these do not cause preterm labor in a normal, low-risk pregnancy.

If you're thinking "mommy" every time you see your wife and her baby-bulge, you may have a harder time getting past your aversion to sexual intimacy. The most important thing is for you both to talk about it and discuss your feelings openly and honestly. Ignoring the problem will breed frustration and anger.

If you do agree to put sex on the back burner for a while, it doesn't mean a moratorium on romance. Bring her flowers, treat her to a weekend getaway, or just cook her dinner one night and spend the evening talking about the future. Above all, enjoy each other and keep your relationship healthy.

Sympathy Pains

Every day she seems to have a new and interesting pregnancy symptom to report. Suddenly, you're feeling them too. Sympathetic pregnancy symptoms, known as couvade, are actually a fairly common occurrence. It's estimated that up to 65 percent of men experience at least one or more pregnancy symptoms during their partner's pregnancy, including nausea, backache, weight gain, and difficulty sleeping. The cause is likely multifaceted—a combination of psychological, social, and possibly even biological factors. They do say that misery loves company; take it as a signal to have some rest and recuperation time together. Ⓔ

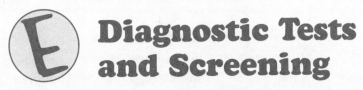

Chapter 5

Diagnostic Tests and Screening

Y ou'll be poked, prodded, swabbed, scraped, and scanned throughout your pregnancy. All these tests have a purpose, of course—a healthy mom and baby. This chapter gives you a rundown of what you have to look forward to and what it all means.

The Basics

At each visit to your provider, you'll have your blood pressure and weight checked and any swelling assessed. Overall, blood pressure tends to go down in pregnancy because of the increase in blood volume, a more elastic cardiovascular system, and other factors. A normal blood pressure range in pregnancy is around 120 (systolic) over 70 (diastolic). Anything higher than 140 over 90 (written 140/90) is considered high. However, hypertension can occur at lower numbers as well. If your systolic pressure rises more than 30 mm over your normal rate (called your baseline), and your diastolic rises more than 15 mm, it may be an early sign of pregnancy-induced hypertension or preeclampsia.

Your belly will be examined. Just how depends on where you are in your pregnancy, but you might expect a regular measurement of your fundal height (the top of your uterus) starting sometime in the second trimester, and an external check of the baby's position in the third trimester.

Finally, at your initial visit, and again in the ninth month when labor approaches, you might have an internal, or pelvic, exam. You're probably familiar with these from your annual gynecological exams, but if you aren't, it's fairly straightforward. A speculum, a duck-billed instrument, is inserted into your vagina and opened to form a tube through which your provider can view your vagina and cervix. It isn't painful, but you will probably experience some pressure that you may consider uncomfortable. He will also scrape off some cervical cells for a Pap smear and take a swab of vaginal fluid to test for sexually transmitted diseases. These also should not hurt.

If you are having a vaginal birth, toward the very end of pregnancy your doctor or midwife will again do an internal, this time to check the cervix for ripening—a sign of approaching labor. For more on cervical ripening, see Chapter 17.

Urine Tests

You'll be giving a urine sample at each prenatal visit for urinalysis. Your provider's office or lab will test your urine for ketones, protein, and glucose at each visit, and may also check for the presence of any bacteria.

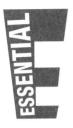

Depending on the protocol followed in your provider's office, you may be asked to either bring a fresh urine specimen to your appointment, or provide one upon your arrival. In either case, it's a good excuse to get some of those extra fluids your body and baby need right now. Down a bottle of drinking water on the way to your checkup so you can easily provide a sample, but don't overdo it or you may not make it without a pit stop.

Ketones

Ketone bodies are substances produced when the body is getting insufficient fuel from food intake and has to metabolize fat for energy. The result is a process known as ketosis, and the resulting ketones spill into the urine. Ketones may appear in pregnancy if you're suffering from severe nausea and vomiting, and they are a sign that you may require intravenous nutrition. They can also be a byproduct of gestational diabetes when blood sugars get too high (above 200 mg/dl), and can lead to a potential life-threatening complication called diabetic ketoacidosis (DKA).

The ketone test is generally performed with a reagent test strip, where a strip of chemically treated paper is dipped in your urine sample and then matched against a color chart for the presence of ketones. Test strips allow your provider or her staff to get fairly instantaneous results.

If you have gestational diabetes, you will probably be prescribed a vial of ketone strips (Ketostix) for home use. Your provider will instruct you in their proper use. Chapter 13 has further information on gestational diabetes and DKA.

Protein

Excessive protein (albumin) in the urine can be a sign of preeclampsia (also known as toxemia or pregnancy induced hypertension). It is also a possible indication of urinary tract infection (UTI) or renal (kidney) impairment. The presence of white blood cells in urine can be an indication of infection as well.

Your provider will again use a test strip to check for protein. If the strip is positive, it indicates that protein levels above 30 mg/dl are detected, which is considered more than the trace amount normally present in urine. A positive protein strip is an indication for further testing with the more specific 24-hour urine test.

In a 24-hour urine test, you'll be given a special container to collect your urine in, and you'll be asked to keep the sample refrigerated during the collection period (which ought to do wonders for your appetite). In a nonpregnant woman, 150 milligrams of total protein excreted in a day is considered normal; pregnant women typically excrete more and a normal test in pregnancy is 260 milligrams or less for a 24-hour period.

If preeclampsia is suspected, your provider will probably order additional tests, including a blood draw, ultrasound, and fetal monitoring. See Chapter 13 for more on this condition.

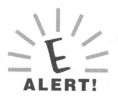
ALERT!

The kidneys are responsible for filtering waste products and fluids from the bloodstream and into urine. Their function is also closely tied to blood pressure regulation. As the volume of fluid in the bloodstream goes up with a blood pressure increase (hypertension), the kidneys must work double time to clean and filter the blood. Eventually, the skyrocketing blood pressure threatens to damage the nephrons (filtering units of the kidneys) and the kidneys in turn cause the blood pressure to rise even further because they aren't able to adequately clear fluids. Be familiar with the warning signs of preeclampsia, which are covered in Chapter 13 of this book.

Glucose

Glucose, or sugar, in the urine (called glycosuria) may be a sign of gestational diabetes mellitus (GDM). It's normal to spill a small amount of sugar into the urine in pregnancy, but consistent high levels along with other risk factors raise a red flag that GDM may be present. Again, test reagent strips (i.e., Diastix, Clinistix) are used for screening. If your doctor suspects GDM, she will order a glucose challenge test (GCT). If this is abnormal, she'll then order an oral glucose tolerance test (GTT; see "Blood Work" following).

Urine Culture

Your urine will be analyzed and cultured for the presence of bacteria at your first prenatal visit, and again during pregnancy if symptoms of a urinary tract infection (e.g., burning during urination, strong smelling urine) appear.

Blood Work

You won't be handing out your blood as frequently as your urine, but there still are a few blood tests involved in pregnancy.

Hemoglobin Count

Your hemoglobin levels, the red blood cells that carry oxygen throughout your body, will be assessed at your initial prenatal visit and may be tested again in the second and third trimesters. Low hemoglobin levels, called anemia, occur frequently in pregnancy due to the vast boost of your total blood volume product. Levels that are too low can be a risk factor for low birth weight babies. If your total hemoglobin levels are below 12 mg/dl, your provider may prescribe iron supplements to build your hemoglobin reserves and order regular hemoglobin screenings at each prenatal visit to monitor your progress.

Glucose Challenge

The glucose challenge test is a screening tool for gestational diabetes mellitus (GDM). It's typically given between 24 and 28 weeks of pregnancy, but may be administered earlier in women considered at risk for GDM.

You may be instructed to carbo load before the test, and then will be given 50 grams of a glucose solution, usually what is known as Glucola, to drink. One hour later, blood will be drawn and your blood serum glucose levels will be measured. A level greater than 135–140 mg/dl is considered high, in which case further testing will be necessary.

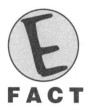

FACT

Some women find that their queasy stomachs simply can't tolerate Glucola—the sugary drink given for gestational diabetes screening. Two separate clinical studies published in the *American Journal of Obstetrics and Gynecology* have shown that a tastier alternative—jelly beans—are an effective stand-in for Glucola for women who experience side effects with the glucose solution.

Oral Glucose Tolerance Test (GTT)

Women who test with high serum glucose levels after the glucose challenge are then given an oral glucose tolerance test to make a definitive diagnosis of gestational diabetes. The GTT, or 3-hour glucose challenge, is a fasting test. You will be instructed not to eat after a certain time before taking it (usually midnight the evening before). Since pregnancy and fasting don't mix too well, especially if morning sickness is a problem, the test is typically administered first thing in the morning.

When you arrive at the lab, blood will be taken, then you will be given 100 grams of Glucola to drink. If the fasting didn't make you sick, it's likely this might. Your blood will be drawn at 1-hour intervals until you reach the 3-hour mark. The glucose levels in the blood samples you provide will be analyzed and checked against the diagnostic criteria for GDM.

The American Diabetes Association recommends lab values known as the Carpenter and Coustan scale for interpreting GTT results. A level of 95 mg/dl or higher at the start of the test, 180 mg/dl or higher at 1 hour, 155 mg/dl or higher at 2 hours, and 140 mg/dl or higher at 3 hours is considered elevated. If two or more levels are elevated, a diagnosis of gestational diabetes is given.

Other Blood Tests

Your blood type and rhesus, or Rh, factor will be determined at your first prenatal visit. An Rh factor is either positive or negative. If your Rh is positive, no treatment is necessary. If you are Rh negative, you are at risk for Rh incompatibility with the blood type of your baby. Rh incompatibility occurs when your unborn baby is Rh positive and your Rh negative blood combines with hers. When this happens, your immune system may try to fight off the baby as an intruder, causing serious complications. Receiving RhoGAM will prevent this from happening.

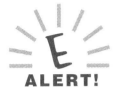

ALERT!

According to the March of Dimes, one in 2,000 women will develop chickenpox during pregnancy. This virus, known clinically as varicella, has the potential to cause birth defects if it is contracted early in pregnancy. Fortunately, there are tests available to determine immunity to varicella, which may be given at the first prenatal appointment if you are unsure if you have ever had the illness. See Chapter 8 for more information.

Blood tests also determine whether or not you are immune to German measles (rubella). German measles can cause birth defects, especially if you contract the infection during the first trimester, and can cause cataracts, heart defects, and deafness in offspring. A majority of women have been exposed to the rubella virus or have been vaccinated against it before becoming pregnant, however, and immunity lasts a lifetime.

An HIV, hepatitis B, or syphilis test may also be done on your blood. For more on the testing of sexually transmitted diseases (STDs), see "Swabs and Smears: Sexually Transmitted Diseases," later in this chapter.

The ACOG now recommends that all pregnant couples, regardless of ethnic background, be offered cystic fibrosis screening. Prior to 2001, only individuals with risk factors for passing along the disease, such as parents of European or Ashkenazi Jewish descent, were typically offered screening. Cystic fibrosis screening is performed on either a blood or saliva sample.

Blood tests can also screen for inherited anemia in at-risk populations. For example, couples of African, Caribbean, Eastern Mediterranean, Middle Eastern, and Asian descent are at risk for sickle cell anemia. Families of Greek, Italian, Turkish, African, West Indian, Arabian, or Asian descent may be screened for the thalassemia trait; if *both* father and mother are carriers, there is a chance that the fetus could develop the blood disease thalassemia major.

The alpha-fetoprotein (AFP) blood tests, or variations called the triple or quad AFP screens, are used in pregnancy to screen for genetic problems and certain birth defects. Page ahead to "Alpha-fetoprotein (AFP)/Triple or Quad Screen Test" for more details.

If initial blood screening tests for genetic conditions are positive, an amniocentesis or CVS can help determine if the trait has been passed on to the baby. A trip to a genetic counselor to weigh all your options and assess their risks and benefits is a good idea.

Swabs and Smears

More bodily fluid tests will be taken throughout pregnancy, particularly at the initial prenatal workup.

Pap Smear

Unless you've had one within the last year, your provider will give you a Pap smear at your initial prenatal visit. During your pelvic exam, she will scrape a small sample of cells from your cervix using a spatula-like instrument. The cells are collected and sent to a lab for microscopic analysis.

An abnormal Pap smear tells your doctor that something is going on with your cervix that requires further examination. While cervical cancer and precancerous spots are a possibility, it is also quite possible that a simple vaginal infection or inflammation of the cervix is behind an abnormal Pap smear. STDs, particularly the human papillomavirus (HPV), can also cause irregularities. A closer look with another pelvic exam should tell your doctor, and you, more.

Group B Strep

Group B streptococcus (GBS) is a bacterium that can cause serious infections in a newborn—including pneumonia and meningitis. If a pregnant woman tests positive for it, she is usually prescribed intravenous antibiotics during labor and delivery to prevent transmission to her baby.

Swabs of both the rectum and vagina are taken and cultured (put in a medium that will allow the bacteria to grow if it is present). The U.S. Centers for Disease Control (CDC) advises that all pregnant women be screened for GBS at 35 to 37 weeks gestation.

Sexually Transmitted Diseases (STDs)

The CDC also recommends that all pregnant women be screened for several sexually transmitted diseases—chlamydia, gonorrhea, hepatitis B, HIV, and syphilis—because of their potentially devastating effects on a fetus. HIV, hepatitis B, and syphilis testing require a blood draw, while chlamydia and gonorrhea are tested with a polymerase chain reaction (PCR) test. You may only be offered some of these tests by your provider based on your medical history and perceived risk factors. If you'd like to be tested for all of them, ask your doctor.

Chlamydia, gonorrhea, and syphilis are caused by bacteria and can be treated with antibiotics. Viral infections like hepatitis B and HIV cannot be cured in the mother, but precautionary measures can greatly decrease the risks of her passing on the disease to her child during labor and delivery.

Ultrasounds

The test that most women look forward to—the ultrasound—gives you your first glimpse at your little one and lets your practitioner assess the baby's growth and development. It may also be used to diagnose placental abnormalities, an ectopic pregnancy, certain birth defects, or other suspected problems.

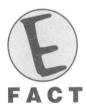

FACT

According to the CDC, over 2.6 million ultrasounds were performed in the United States in 2000. American women also had 96,698 amniocentesis procedures in 2000.

There are two types of ultrasound scans: the transabdominal, which scans through your abdomen, and the transvaginal, which scans directly into your vagina. In very early pregnancy, the technician may opt for the vaginal approach, which means that the transducer will be inserted into your vagina. However, abdominal ultrasounds are the most common as most ultrasounds take place in the second the third trimesters.

An ultrasound typically takes no longer than a half-hour to perform. If you are in the first half of your pregnancy, you will probably be instructed to drink plenty of water prior to the exam, and refrain from emptying your bladder. This is probably the most difficult part of the test. The extra fluids help the technician to visualize your baby.

Once in the examining room, you will recline on a table or bed with your upper body elevated and your abdomen exposed. Ask for extra pillows if you tend to get woozy when not lying on your side. The lights may be dimmed to allow the operator to see the sonogram picture more clearly. A thin application of transducer paste, jelly, or oil will be spread on your abdomen and then the fun begins.

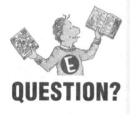

QUESTION?

My doctor has prescribed a level-two ultrasound. Should I be concerned?
A level-two ultrasound uses the same technology as a regular sonogram, but involves a more detailed analysis of the results. It is frequently performed by a perinatologist who is specially trained in its use. The doctor will check fetal growth, organ system development, position of the placenta, and amniotic fluid volume. There are a number of reasons for a level two to be ordered, from the routine to the potentially more serious. Your doctor should keep you informed, so if he hasn't given you a reason, ask.

The ultrasound picture, or sonogram, is obtained when high-frequency sound waves are passed over your abdomen with a hand-held wand called a transducer. These waves bounce off the solid structures of your baby, sending back a moving image of the tiny being inside. The resulting picture is transmitted to a computer or television screen. Ultrasound pictures are typically a grainy black and white, but new three-dimensional ultrasound technologies on the market can display your child in living (but simulated) color and are incredibly lifelike. The two dimensional units are more common, however, in part because they are much less expensive. The ultrasound operator can print out pictures for you to take home, so if she doesn't offer, make sure you ask.

The newest wave in ultrasound—four-dimensional technology—is actually 3-D with movement added. The picture is clearer, and the movement component allows for diagnosis of heart defects. It can also be used to check for markers of developmentally normal fetal movements.

The ultrasound technician may take a series of measurements during the procedure with the computer attached to the machine. These measurements help your provider assess the growth and organ development of the fetus. Depending on the timing of the test and the cooperation of your unborn child, she may also be able to get an idea of his or her gender. Typically, this information won't be given unless you ask for it, in case you prefer to be surprised at birth. Once the test is over, the technician will help you clean the transducer gel off your belly and you'll be able to empty your bladder, if need be.

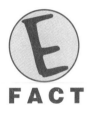

FACT

Although an estimated 70 percent of pregnant women in the United States currently have at least one ultrasound, the ACOG does not currently support routine prenatal ultrasounds in low-risk pregnancies (except for specific medical indications). However, the routine use of ultrasounds is widespread outside of the United States; in Denmark, for example, 90 percent of women are offered a routine sonogram early in the first trimester.

When and if you have an ultrasound will depend upon your provider. Many obstetricians order ultrasounds as a matter of routine. Some do one at the first visit to check for correct dates and viability with the rationale that it may save them from questioning gestational dates later on (as dating is more accurate in the first trimester). Others will recommend a sonogram at around 20 weeks to examine the fetal anatomy and ensure the pregnancy is progressing normally.

A patient's peace of mind may also be reason enough to order an ultrasound. Since it is a noninvasive and fairly inexpensive test that can reassure the parents that things are developing normally, many providers will comply with a woman's request for an ultrasound. If your doctor hasn't ordered one and you have some anxieties about your baby's health, it can't hurt to ask.

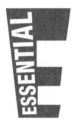

If your fetus isn't feeling coy on ultrasound day, a sonogram taken after 16 weeks may reveal his or her sex. A sighting of a little girl's labia (visible as three parallel lines) or a boy's penis and testicles is necessary to get a fairly positive ID. As a general rule, your technician will probably not commit to an answer on the gender unless she sees one or the other. Just because a penis isn't visible doesn't necessarily mean you have a girl. If you do get a boy or girl answer, keep in mind that barring genetic testing, nothing is 100 percent certain until you meet your "him" or "her" in the delivery room.

Alpha-fetoprotein (AFP)/Triple or Quad Screen Test

Alpha-fetoprotein is a blood protein produced by your unborn baby and passed into your circulatory system. The AFP, administered between weeks 16 and 18, is a blood test used to screen for chromosomal irregularities like trisomy 18 and Down syndrome, and also for neural tube defects. Results of this test are usually available in about a week.

Most of the time, a high level of AFP can be explained by multiple gestation (twins, triplets, or more). However, it could also mean that your fetus has a neural tube defect. If AFP levels are low, it may be an indication of Down syndrome, trisomy 18, or other chromosomal disorders. It could also mean that your dates are wrong. A level-one or level-two ultrasound or an amniocentesis may be ordered for further evaluation. You may also be referred to a genetic counselor.

A more extensive version of the AFP, called the triple-screen test (or AFP-3), measures levels of human chorionic gonadotropin (hCG) and estriol, a type of estrogen, as well as AFP. The quad-test, an even more sensitive marker of chromosomal problems, assesses all three of these substances plus inhibin-A.

A misdated pregnancy can affect the results of your AFP or triple or quad screen and give a false positive. An ultrasound can help to confirm or adjust the gestational age.

Amniocentesis

The thought of an amniocentesis makes many women nervous, probably because it involves two critical undertakings: a needle being inserted through the abdomen and breaching your baby's watery environment. It does carry some risk of complications, including a slight chance of miscarriage. However, the amnio (as it is commonly referred to) is one of the best tools available for diagnosing chromosomal abnormalities, genetic disorders, and birth defects. An amniocentesis is typically performed in the second trimester after week 15 or 16 of pregnancy, although a later amnio may be done depending on the indication (or reason). At this point in pregnancy there are enough fetal cells present in the amniotic fluid for withdrawal and analysis.

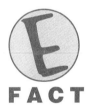

FACT

In addition to the wealth of genetic and health information it provides, an amnio can also tell you definitively if your baby is a boy or a girl. If you want to be surprised about the sex of your child, it may be a good idea to restate your wishes before you receive your amnio results.

Your provider may suggest you meet with a genetic counselor prior to having an amniocentesis performed to weigh the risks versus the benefits of the procedure, given your specific medical background and family history. She will also lay out any alternative procedures that may be options, such as a level-two ultrasound. If you do decide to go with the amnio, you may be sent to a perinatologist, or maternal-fetal specialist, who is experienced in the procedure.

An amniocentesis is a relatively short outpatient procedure. Your abdomen is first swabbed with an antiseptic solution. The physician will use the abdominal ultrasound procedure to see her way around your womb. She will then insert a needle into the amniotic sac and draw an amniotic fluid sample into a syringe. The fluid contains sloughed-off fetal cells, which will be analyzed in the lab.

Here are reasons why an amniocentesis may be planned:

- **Age:** Women over 35 have an increased risk of carrying a baby with a chromosomal disorder like Down syndrome When the father is over fifty, amniocentesis could also be advised because there may be a connection between paternal age and an increased risk of Down syndrome.
- **Family history:** If you've already had a baby with a hereditary or chromosomal abnormality or neural tube defects, an amniocentesis could make you feel more comfortable.
- **Rh status:** Rh negative women may have an amnio to determine the Rh status of their fetus.
- **AFP, triple screen, or quad-test results:** If alpha-fetoprotein (AFP) shows up at a higher than normal level, an amnio may help clear up any questions.
- **Ultrasound abnormalities:** If your ultrasound turned up indications of the possibility of a chromosomal disorder, an amnio may be recommended for further evaluation.
- **Lung maturity:** If you're experiencing symptoms of preterm labor or other medical complications that point to an early birth, your provider may perform an amnio to check the level of surfactant present in the fluid, a marker of fetal lung maturity.
- **Infection:** If you have preterm labor and your doctor is worried about an infection, an amnio may be recommended.

After the amnio procedure, the baby will be monitored by ultrasound and will have his heart rate checked for a few minutes to ensure that everything is okay. You may experience minimal cramping. You will be advised to restrict strenuous exercise for one day (no step aerobics), although other normal activity should be fine. If in the days following amnio you experience fluid or blood discharge from the vagina, let your provider know as soon as possible.

The U.S. Centers for Disease Control and Prevention (CDC) estimates the chance of miscarriage following an amnio at somewhere between one in 400 and one in 200, and the risk of uterine infection at less than one in 1,000. There is also a slight risk of trauma to the unborn baby from a misplaced needle or inadvertent rupture of the sac.

If there are problems, the information you get from an amnio can prepare you for providing your child with the best care possible at birth. However, the timing can make other decisions difficult. Results from your amniocentesis won't be available for up to 2 weeks. And by the time the test results are back, you will be halfway through your pregnancy (about 20 weeks). For this reason, some women at risk for chromosomal abnormalities will choose the chorionic villus sampling test, which can be performed in the first trimester, instead.

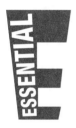

Some studies suggest that the experience and associated skill level of the physician performing a CVS or amniocentesis can make a big difference in the risk of complications. Many physicians will refer you to a perinatologist or other specialist for just this reason. If your provider is performing the procedure, feel free to ask for an estimate of how many amnios or CVS procedures she has under her belt.

Chorionic Villus Sampling (CVS)

CVS stands for chorionic villus sampling, a test performed in the first trimester (usually between weeks 10 and 12) to assess chromosomal abnormalities and hereditary conditions in the unborn baby. Your provider will use ultrasound guidance to insert a catheter into the placenta, either through the cervix (transcervical) or through a needle injected into the abdomen (transabdominal). The catheter is used to extract a biopsy (or sample) of the tiny chorionic villi, the fingers of tissue surrounding the embryo that are the beginnings of the placenta. The villi are a genetic match for the baby's own tissue.

Slight cramping and spotting is normal after the procedure, and you will probably be advised to indulge in some rest and relaxation for the remainder of the day. If bleeding continues, is excessive, or is accompanied by pain or fever, call your practitioner immediately.

CVS has several benefits over amnio. It can be performed earlier (first trimester as opposed to second) and the results are available much faster (5 to 7 days for preliminary CVS results versus 10 to 14 days for amnio). However, the risk of miscarriage is higher with CVS—between 1 in 200 and 1 in 100 will experience miscarriage after the procedure. The risk is higher for woman with a retroverted (tipped, or tilted) uterus who are given a transcervical CVS (about 5 in 100). For this reason, a transabdominal CVS (through the abdominal wall) is usually advised for these women. A consultation with a genetic counselor can help you analyze the positives and negatives and decide if a CVS is right for you.

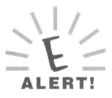

ALERT!

A CVS is not always accurate. The exact spot where the technician removes the cell sampling from the chorion can be critical. Also, some abnormalities in chorionic tissues do not always show up in the fetus. Ask for clarification or a second opinion of any negative CVS report before you decide on any course of action in your pregnancy.

Fetal Monitoring

A fetal heart monitor measures—you guessed it—the fetal heart rate (or FHR). A baseline, or average, fetal heart rate of 120 to 160 beats per minute (bpm) is considered normal. Spikes as high as 25 bpm are normal and coincide with fetal stimulation and sleep cycles.

During Labor

Fetal monitors also measure the length and severity of contractions. There are both external and internal monitors available. An external monitor uses two belts that are positioned around your belly. The transducers on each are adjusted until they are both measuring your contractions and picking up the fetal heart sounds.

If you are in a high-risk pregnancy, you may be hooked up to an internal fetal monitor during labor and delivery. Internal monitors may only be used in labor when the amniotic sac has broken. This monitor is considered more sensitive and accurate, but is also more invasive. It uses a little spring-like wire that is inserted vaginally and sits just under the skin on the baby's head.

Both internal and external monitoring can keep you tethered to your bed during labor, which may not be the experience you want. External monitors, however, can be removed for a short time, but in general fetal movement should be assessed at least every 15 minutes. A new type of monitor that uses telemetry allows some women to go wireless for labor. For more on telemetry, see Chapter 18.

Stress and Non-Stress Test (NST)

If there is any concern about fetal well-being or if you are still waiting for baby's belated arrival at 41 or 42 weeks, you'll probably be given a non-stress test. A non-stress test (NST) measures fetal heart rate and is performed any time after 24 weeks. When you move, your heart rate speeds up, and when baby moves, his heart rate speeds up, the sign of a healthy fetus.

The test is administered on a bed or examining table attached to a fetal monitor (see above). The monitor belts are strapped around your abdomen. For about 20 minutes, every time you feel your baby move, you'll push a button. The button will record the movement on the paper strip or computer record of baby's heartbeat. Depending on how the monitor is hooked up, it may also detect and note the movement. Rises in the FHR should correspond to fetal movement.

If there is no movement, it's quite possible that baby is sleeping. You'll be given a drink of juice or small snack in an attempt to rouse her. Sometimes, a buzzer or vibrations called vibroacoustic stimulation are used to wake up a sleeping fetus. If these methods are unsuccessful, further testing is needed, and a biophysical profile (BPP) may be ordered. Fifteen percent of NSTs before 32 weeks are nonreactive.

In a stress test (also called a contraction stress test [CST] or oxytocin challenge test), mild contractions are induced with the hormone Pitocin to see how your baby responds. You will be hooked up to a fetal monitor and you will receive a Pitocin (oxytocin) injection. If the baby cannot maintain his heartbeat during a contraction, immediate delivery may be indicated (possibly by C-section).

Biophysical Profile (BPP)

A biophysical profile (BPP) is simply an ultrasound combined with a non-stress test (NST). A BPP assesses fetal heart rate, muscle tone, body and breathing movement, and the amount of amniotic fluid, which are all noted and included on your chart. The test takes about a half hour, and a score of 8 to 10 is normal. A low BPP score may indicate that the fetus is getting insufficient oxygen. If the fetal lungs are mature, immediate delivery may be recommended.

Women in high-risk pregnancies may undergo regular weekly or biweekly BPP testing in the third trimester. BPP is also a standard test for a post-term pregnancy that has gone beyond 42 weeks. Your physician may also order a modified biophysical profile, which is a BPP that consists of the NST and an ultrasound assessment of amniotic fluid (the amniotic fluid index, or AFI) only.

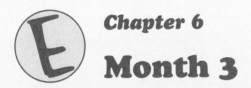

Chapter 6

Month 3

This is a landmark month as you finish up your first trimester! You start to sport a protruding belly, which may mean sharing your news with friends, family, and coworkers if you haven't already. Your little fetus is growing by leaps and bounds, and you make first contact this month as you hear her heartbeat and perhaps even see her on ultrasound.

Baby This Month

By the end of this month, baby will grow to over 3 inches in length and almost one ounce, about the size and heft of a roll of Lifesavers. If you could look at his face, you'd see that his ears and closed eyelids have now fully developed. His head accounts for one-third of his total length, and his tongue, salivary glands, and taste buds have also formed. Even though he's a long way from his first meal, studies indicate he may already be getting a taste of what you've been snacking on from the maternal blood supply or placenta.

He is now getting all of his nutrients through the fully formed placenta (from the Greek *plakous*, meaning flat cake, its approximately shape), an organ that you and your fetus share. The umbilical cord tethers the fetus to the placenta, which provides it with nutrients and oxygen and transports waste materials away.

Your baby's heart is pumping about 25 quarts of blood each day, and a lattice of blood vessels can be seen through his translucent skin, which is starting to develop a coat of fine downy hair called lanugo. His, or her, gender is apparent since the external sex organs have now fully differentiated, but it will take a combination of luck and technical skill for an ultrasound operator to reveal if you have a son or daughter. (For more on ultrasound exams, see Chapter 5.)

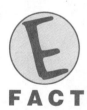

FACT

While 15 to 20 percent of pregnancies result in miscarriage in the first trimester, by the time you hear your baby's heartbeat around week 12, the risk of miscarriage for most women has dropped to only 3 percent.

Your Body This Month

You probably never thought you'd be pleased by a potbellied profile, but this significant, visible sign of your pregnancy is a landmark moment for many women. Wear it proudly. You've taken your child through the first 3 critical months of growth, and your belly is a badge of honor that tells the world about this important accomplishment.

Your Body Changes

Your uterus is about the size of a softball and stretches to just about your pubic bone. About 2 to 4 pounds of total weight gain is average for the first trimester; if you've been down and out with nausea and vomiting, you may be below the curve. Weight gain will pick up in the second trimester and peak in the third as your baby starts to fill out your womb.

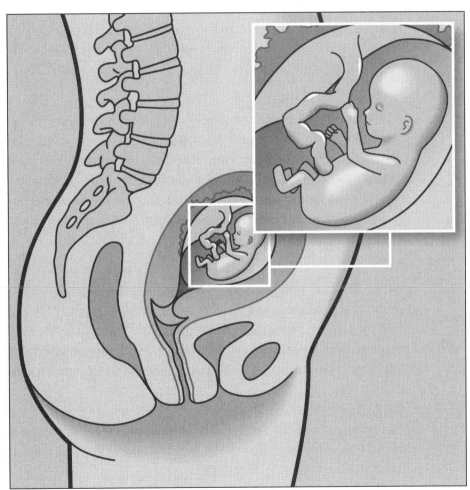

▲ You and your fetus at the end of the first trimester.

Don't take the "eating for two" cliché literally—300 extra calories per day is about all you'll require to meet your baby's nutritional needs.

Gaining too much can exacerbate the aches and pains of pregnancy, place an extra strain on your back, and may put you at risk for hypertension (high blood pressure) problems.

At the same time, if you find the aversions and nausea of pregnancy have you only keeping down a certain type of not-so-nutritious food (pepperoni pizza, for example), don't feel bad about it. The most important thing right now is keeping food down and your energy up. Try experimenting with some healthier variations if your stomach will take it (skip the pepperoni in exchange for extra cheese or veggies), and hang in there. By the end of the first trimester most women report that their morning sickness gets better or (fingers crossed) completely disappears.

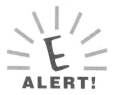

ALERT!

The FDA advises pregnant women to eat no more than 12 ounces of cooked fish (canned, fresh, or frozen) each week, and to steer clear of shark, swordfish, king mackerel, and tilefish completely. Although packed with protein and nutrients, fish, especially larger fish like these four species, may contain high levels of mercury, which can hamper development of your baby's central nervous system.

While 25 to 35 pounds is the average suggested total weight gain for a pregnancy, your height and build will influence that number. Underweight women and women with multiple pregnancies (twins or more) will be expected to gain more, overweight women will be encouraged to gain slightly less. If your provider hasn't mentioned a weight goal for your pregnancy, ask him what his expectations are.

Most important, don't let the scale become an obsession. Focus instead on the quality of food you're eating and on getting some regular exercise (cleared with your provider first). Your health, and baby's health, is the ultimate goal of this pregnancy.

Breakdown of where the weight goes
Baby—7.5 to 8.5 pounds
Uterus—2 to 2.5 pounds

Breakdown of where the weight goes *(cont'd)*

Placenta—1.5 to 2 pounds

Amniotic fluid—2 pounds

Blood—3 to 4 pounds

Breasts—1 to 2 pounds

Maternal fat and nutrient stores—4 to 6 pounds

Retained maternal fluids—4 to 8 pounds

What You Feel Like

Although nausea and vomiting may finally be waning thanks to a decline in hCG levels, constipation, gas, and occasional heartburn may take over as the gastrointestinal pests of the next trimester. Constipation is caused by an increase in progesterone, which can act to slow down the digestive system. Later in the pregnancy, pressure on the intestine caused by your growing uterus adds to the problem.

Iron supplements or prenatal vitamins with added iron can also cause constipation, so talking to your provider about the possibility of a dosage adjustment or an extended release formula may be in order. An increase in dietary fiber, plenty of water intake, and exercise as approved by your health care provider may also help to get things going again. Be sure to consult your doctor before taking any stool softeners or laxatives.

Gas may become a source of discomfort and occasional embarrassment as well. Consider cutting back on foods that worsen the problem (e.g., onions, beans, broccoli, cabbage, carbonated drinks). Fiber you take to eliminate constipation can also aggravate gas problems. Try small, frequent snacks instead of large meals to keep the burps at bay.

Other pregnancy symptoms that may continue or begin this month include:

- Fatigue
- Frequent urination
- Tender breasts
- Nausea

- Headaches
- Increased saliva
- Nasal congestion and/or runny nose
- Occasional dizziness or faintness

At the Doctor

Make sure your husband or partner makes this month's prenatal appointment. You're both in for a treat as you begin to experience the sights and sounds of your growing child.

Tests This Month

Depending on your provider's policy on ultrasound exams and your personal medical history, you may be seeing your baby this month. For the complete story on ultrasound examinations, please see Chapter 5.

Your provider will also start estimating the size of your baby by taking a tape measure to your belly and counting the centimeters from your pubic bone to the tip of your fundus—the top of the uterus. Taking this measurement at each visit gives your practitioner a way to assess your baby's ongoing growth. Some practitioners do not take the fundal height until after week 12 or even week 20.

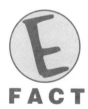

FACT

Variances in fundal height could indicate problems such as gestational diabetes or intrauterine growth retardation. At 20 weeks, the length should be equivalent to the baby's gestational age, give or take 3 centimeters. However, fundal height is used as a screening tool only; women who are overweight, carrying multiples, or have a fetus in the breech position may not measure accurately.

You may be told about the alpha-fetoprotein test this month. The AFP is typically given at 16 to 18 weeks, and tests for the possibility of neural tube defects and/or chromosomal abnormalities in the fetus. Since it is optional, many providers give an informational sheet to patients the month before so they have time to consider whether they want to take it. For more on the AFP test, see Chapter 5.

Baby's Heartbeat

Hearing the steady "woosh-woosh" of your baby's heart for the first time is one of the most thrilling and emotional moments of pregnancy.

Your chance at first contact happens this month as your provider checks for the fetal heartbeat using a small ultrasound device called a Doppler or Doptone. If you have a retroverted uterus (also known as a tipped or tilted uterus), it's possible the Doppler won't detect the heartbeat just yet. Don't be alarmed; by your next prenatal appointment you will probably be able to hear her loud and clear.

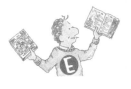

QUESTION?

I've reached the magic 15-week mark and I'm still sick as a dog. Could I be having twins?
While lingering and/or excessive nausea and vomiting in pregnancy can indicate twins, in the absence of other signs of multiples it's more likely a simple matter of your unique body chemistry and pregnancy. Hang in there, talk to your provider, and try some of the morning sickness suggestions in Chapter 2. (For more on multiple pregnancies, see Chapter 7.)

On Your Mind

Feel like you're losing your mind while gaining three dress sizes? Coping with forgetfulness and learning to love your changing body are just a few of the issues facing you as you close out the first trimester.

Forgetfulness

Have you walked around looking for your sunglasses for 20 minutes before finding them on your head? Lost your car keys for the fifth time this week? Like any mom-to-be, you've got a lot on your mind. That alone may have you forgetting what used to be second nature and misplacing things. Although researchers have looked at the problem of memory impairment in pregnancy, there hasn't been a clear consensus on what the definitive cause is. Pregnancy hormones, sleep deprivation, and stress have all been suggested as possible culprits. A 2002 study published in the *Journal of Reproductive Medicine* found that women in their second trimester of pregnancy who reported memory problems had lower blood levels of the neurotransmitters norepinephrine, epinephrine, and serotonin than their nonpregnant peers, suggesting that these brain chemicals may somehow be related to memory loss.

Whatever the cause, forgetting appointments and misplacing things can leave you feeling muddled and helpless. Try relying less on your memory by writing notes, sticking to a routine (e.g., car keys always go into a basket by the door), and living by a written or electronic organizer. If you aren't the Palm Pilot type, start requesting a 24-hour advance phone call reminder when you schedule service appointments such as in-home appliance repair or a salon appointment. Having a system—whatever it is—is the key to staying reasonably organized and mentally together during this hectic time.

Feeling Good about Your Changing Body

A word on weight—try not to get too hung up on it. Stepping on the scale at every doctor's visit may make weight seem like a pass or fail test, but it is just one tool your provider has to make sure your baby is growing on schedule. Don't dread the regular weigh-in—look at what it tells you as tangible proof your unborn child is growing and developing well.

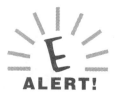

ALERT!

Never diet in pregnancy, even if you've already gained more than expected. Restricting calorie and nutrient intake can hamper fetal development. If you're concerned about excessive weight gain, consider seeing a registered dietitian for help with meal planning and/or taking a provider-approved prenatal exercise class.

Don't compare yourself to those who have gone before you, as well. If older neighbors, friends, and relatives remark on their own minimal weight gain and quick return to prepregnancy weight, there's a reason. Up through the 1970s, "ideal" pregnancy weight gains averaged 10 to 15 pounds less than they do today, according to the Institute of Medicine. Studies have since shown that weight gain should be individualized to a mother's prepregnancy body mass index (BMI), and that inadequate weight gain can contribute to low birth-weight babies.

Now is a good time to go out and buy that first maternity outfit if you haven't already done so. Pick out something comfortable and stylish that makes you feel good, and maybe even shows off your belly a bit.

Spreading the Word

Now that you're showing, keeping your pregnancy to yourself will be increasingly difficult. If you and your partner have kept the good news to yourself so far—for a whole trimester no less—now is probably the time to spill it.

Sharing with Friends and Family

How you tell your parents, siblings, and best friends that you and your partner are pregnant can be one of the most exciting parts of pregnancy. It can also be a little nerve-wracking if you're not sure how the news will be received.

If you've held off sharing your pregnancy until now, "Why did you wait so long to tell us?!?" may be a common refrain. Whatever your reasons for waiting are, they're valid. Let your family and friends know that they're important to you, which is why you've chosen to make them among the first outside of you and your partner to know about your new addition.

Some fun ideas for sharing the news with parents, friends, or others:

- Give them an ultrasound picture (or a photocopy of one), and let it explain itself.
- Send out birthday invitations for the estimated due date.
- Take out a "Help Wanted: Grandparents" advertisement in their local classifieds and point them to it.
- Invite them to dinner (at home or out) and serve a frosting-inscribed "It's a Boy/Girl/Fetus," "Congratulations Auntie," or "We're Pregnant" cake for dessert.
- Ask your mom or sister to go shopping with you and take her to your 3-month ob/gyn appointment instead.
- If this isn't your first, let your kids spread the news in their own

special way.

• The old standby—"Guess what?"—works well too.

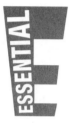

Alas, there are some people in the world who are perpetually in the glass-half-empty state of mind. You may be related to one of them. If you expect a negative reaction from someone that must be clued in on the pregnancy (read: immediate family member), try to take along your spouse or partner for emotional support. Hopefully, the wet blanket will surprise you both with a hug and well wishes. If not, treat yourself to a date with your spouse and let it go as a character defect—theirs.

When (and What) to Tell Work

Now that your pregnancy is becoming more visible and your doctor's appointments are taking you away from the office on a regular basis, it may be a good time to let your employer in on your secret. From a practical viewpoint, you'll want to find out about your company's leave policy, maternity benefits, and health insurance coverage for new family members.

So how do you break the news? Make sure you tell your supervisor or manager first. Hearing about your impending maternity leave through the grapevine may make your manager question your future commitment to your career. Go into the meeting with an idea of how much maternity leave you'd like to take, and even better, who might cover your job responsibilities while you're away.

If you're asked about your plans after baby is born, be honest while playing your cards close to your vest. If you're happy with your career and workplace but unsure whether your tune will change once you see your darling son or daughter, let your employer know you have every intention of returning to work and leave it at that. Disingenuous? Not at all. You can't give a definite response on something that hasn't even occurred yet. That's like asking your employer to make a hiring decision on an applicant he hasn't interviewed yet. You can, however, give him your assurances that you're pleased with your position, if that's the case.

On the other hand, if you've already decided that motherhood will be your new full-time vocation, quitting right after your maternity leave runs out with no fair warning to your supervisor is a sure-fire way to burn bridges and ruin references. Check out your spouse's health insurance and see if you can be switched over to it now so you can give your employer ample notice to find a replacement. If you're worried about losing your job before you're ready, let your supervisor know how long you'd like to work and point out the advantages of using the time to have you train your replacement.

For more on working through and beyond pregnancy, see Chapter 9.

Just for Dads

A boy to bond with or a girl to graduate magna cum laude from Harvard? You and your significant other may be thinking about the prospect of a son or daughter, especially if you have an ultrasound appointment approaching. If you're going to try and find out the gender of your child, keep an open mind since you have little choice in the matter. Think instead of the exceptional beauties and joys to be found in both sexes, and the special sibling relationships to be forged both between and among brothers and sisters. More importantly, start thinking of your baby in terms of potential rather than gender-imposed limitations—girls can carry on the family name just as readily as boys.

Speaking of names, you have probably already started to think about names for the little one. Below are the most popular names for babies born in 2002.

The 10 most popular U.S. baby names for 2002			
Boys' Names		**Girls' Names**	
1. Jacob	6. Joseph	1. Emily	6. Ashley
2. Michael	7. Andrew	2. Madison	7. Abigail
3. Joshua	8. Christopher	3. Hannah	8. Sarah
4. Matthew	9. Daniel	4. Emma	9. Samantha
5. Ethan	10. Nicholas	5. Alexis	10. Olivia

Source: U.S. Social Security Administration

The Cost of Kids

Worried about how to make ends meet as your family grows? First, read our Chapter 3 tips on financial planning and paying for pregnancy. Then, sit down with your significant other and work through a budget together. Chances are there's a lot of room for cutting back, and a lot of things—like movies, concerts, and those weekend getaways—that you won't be doing, or paying for, anymore (at least until your child is a little older).

Still concerned that you won't bring home enough to support your family? You might look at pregnancy as a new beginning for you as well. If you've been thinking about making a career move, spiff up your resume and network now while things are still relatively quiet in your household. Even if you really love your job, finding out what else is out there and getting an offer on the table can give you leverage for negotiating with your current employer.

Changing Roles

You, a dad? The same guy whose idea of a savings account is 6 month's worth of bar change in a water cooler bottle? The same guy who still collects *Star Wars* action figures ("ahem—that's *collectibles*")? The same guy who still calls his dad when the car acts up and who has 20 more years of student loan payments ahead of him? It's hard to grasp until you actually experience it, but the responsibilities, intense love, and fierce protectiveness that are part of parenthood will make you feel more "adult" than just about any event in your life thus far. Believe it or not, some day that little boy or girl will be calling you for automotive advice (and playing with your collectibles). Ⓔ

Chapter 7

Multiple Choice: Two, Three, Four, or More

News of impending twins, triplets, and other multiple gestations is certainly a thrilling, and momentous, surprise for any couple. Disbelief, distinction, and panic are just a few of the feelings you might experience on the road to parenting multiples.

Splitting Eggs and Sharing Sacs

Multiples are either monozygotic (formed from a single egg and sperm) or dizygotic (formed from two separate eggs and sperm). Monozygotic multiples, more commonly known as "identicals," can be further classified by the way they share their common space and maternal resources.

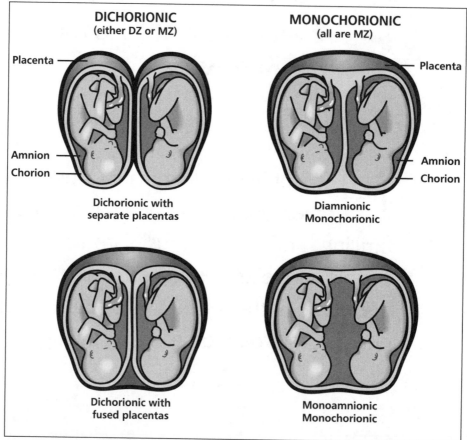

DICHORIONIC
(either DZ or MZ)

MONOCHORIONIC
(all are MZ)

Placenta

Placenta

Amnion

Amnion

Chorion

Chorion

Dichorionic with
separate placentas

Diamnionic
Monochorionic

Dichorionic with
fused placentas

Monoamnionic
Monochorionic

▲ Monozygotic, or identical, twins may each have its own set of fetal membranes, or they may share an amniotic sac (monoamniotic), a chorion membrane (monochorionic), or both.

Identical Twins

Identical, or monozygotic, twins form when a single fertilized egg (zygote) splits in two. Because they are cut from the same piece of genetic fabric, they are always the same gender. Monozygotic twins also share a placenta. Depending on when the zygote splits, they may share an amniotic sac and/or the chorionic membrane, or they may each have their own personal space and membranes. Twins that split more than 1 week after fertilization will probably share both the amnion and the chorion, while twins that split early on are more likely to have separate quarters.

A single zygote that produces twins usually splits within days of fertilization, but may wait up to 2 weeks. Zygotes that split beyond 14 days increase the risk of resulting in conjoined twins, or twins who haven't separated completely and develop with shared body parts or organ systems. Fraternal twins, because they start life as two eggs fertilized by two sperms, do not run the risk of conjoinment.

Fraternal Multiples

Fraternal, or dizygotic, twins are basically siblings in the womb. Each one is created from a separate egg fertilized with its own sperm. Fraternal twins are three times more common than identical twins. They have their own placentas, can be the same or different genders, and may not look any more alike than siblings born individually.

Who Has Multiples?

Your chances of "twinning" are actually not bad—about 1 in 90 births result in twins. If fraternal twins run in your family, your odds are slightly higher. The number of twins and multiple births has skyrocketed over the past several decades, and the incidence of higher order multiples—which include triplets, quadruplets, or more—grew a whopping 404 percent between 1980 and 1997, but has experienced a slow but steady decline since 1999. Twins are more common then ever, however, with 119,648 twin births occurring in 2000.

Why the bonus baby boom? The CDC attributes approximately two-thirds of all U.S. higher order multiples to the use of fertility treatments, also known as assisted reproductive technology (ART). Over 37 percent of all successful pregnancies from ART result in a multiple fraternal birth.

National statistics also reveal that more women are waiting until their thirties and forties to have children, and the increasing twin rate may reflect that reality. Women over 35, especially those who have had a previous multiple birth, have an increased chance of having multiples.

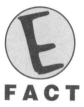

FACT

While birth outcomes of a singleton pregnancy involve more risk as maternal age increases, researchers at the National Institute of Child Health and Human Development (NICHD) and University of Kansas have found that the opposite seems to hold true for multiples pregnancies among older moms. In fact, their 2002 study comparing birth outcomes in triplet pregnancies found that moms over 35 had healthier babies with fewer complications than younger triplet moms. This is probably due in part to the increased use of ART in older women, and the fact that ART multiples rarely share the same amniotic sac—a risk factor for a number of prenatal complications in multiples pregnancies.

Your Body in Multiples Pregnancy

You are living larger than you ever imagined. With all those arms and legs flailing about, you feel as if you're housing a team of tiny Olympic hopefuls. Although it may not feel like it when your crowd is going wild and your back is killing you, a multiples pregnancy is a truly unique gift. That your body can accommodate and nurture not just one, but two, three, or possibly more human beings is nothing short of miraculous.

Moms-to-be of multiples experience the same pregnancy symptoms as women with only one fetus, but they may be more intense and occur earlier in the pregnancy. Excessive nausea and vomiting, in particular, is often an early sign that your unborn child has company. However, many women with singleton pregnancies can experience severe morning sickness as well. More significant markers of multiple pregnancies would include the presence of more than one fetal heart tone during a prenatal examination and measuring too large for your suspected gestational age after week 24.

High levels of alpha-fetoprotein (AFP) on an AFP, triple-screen, or quad-screen blood test may also be an indication that you have some stowaways. For more on AFP, see Chapter 5.

Doctor's Visits

If you've been diagnosed with a multiple pregnancy, you'll be visiting your doctor more frequently. Your appointment schedule will depend on your specific medical history and risk factors involved with your pregnancy, but you might be making the visit twice monthly in early pregnancy (as opposed to just a monthly visit for the first trimester with singleton pregnancies), until you shift to weekly visits early in the third trimester.

Diagnosis

While a number of symptoms and screening tests may point to a multiple pregnancy, a definitive diagnosis is usually made by ultrasound. During the ultrasound procedure, the technician will try to determine whether or not the fetuses are sharing a single amniotic sac since this may put them at higher risk for some complications.

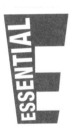

Other moms of twins or multiples can be a great source of information, support, and advice for the unique issues you face, both during pregnancy and after birth. You don't have to stake out the local parks looking for twins; a local or regional "parents of multiples club" can put you in touch with someone in your area. Appendix A includes resources for "multiples moms-to-be."

Do You Need a Perinatalogist?

A perinatologist, an ob-gyn that specializes in high-risk pregnancies, is a good choice for many women expecting multiples. If your medical history is complicated, or if you are expecting triplets or more, the expertise of a perinatologist could be quite valuable. When choosing a perinatologist, it should again be someone you feel comfortable and able to communicate with. There may be a specialist in the practice your original doctor or midwife belongs to, who can make the transition easier. See Chapter 1 for more on choosing a provider that's right for you.

If you decide against a specialist, talk with your provider about his experience delivering multiples, his caesarean rate for this type of birth, and his planned course of action for your specific case. In some cases, your provider may feel that your medical history warrants a referral to a perinatologist, who has a higher level of expertise to handle your pregnancy and delivery, but he may be willing to continue seeing you in conjunction with your specialist for prenatal care.

Problems in Multiple Pregnancies

Multiple pregnancies have a shorter gestation time than singleton pregnancies, simply because there just isn't enough room and resources in mom to house the brood for 40 weeks. Full term for a twin pregnancy is considered 38 weeks (triplets are full term at 35 weeks and quads at 34 weeks). The biggest risk by far in a multiples pregnancy is preterm labor and premature birth.

Problems Mom May Face

If your body is nourishing two or more children, you need to treat it with a little extra TLC. Take an additional 600 calories daily of healthy foods (beyond average prepregnancy calorie intake), and drink plenty of water. The latter is particularly important since dehydration can trigger preterm contractions.

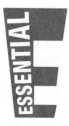

Although due dates are typically based on a 10 lunar month calendar, most people consider pregnancy a 9-month, 3-trimester affair. That's why you'll find your pregnancy divided into 9 calendar months in this book. (For more on estimating your due date, see Chapter 2.)

Moms-to-be of multiples are at greater risk for developing anemia and should speak to their provider about iron supplementation to ensure that their needs are covered. Increasing your intake of iron-rich foods is a good way to ward off anemia. Try rotating iron-fortified foods such as baked beans, black strap molasses, wheat germ, raisins, beef, and leafy green veggies (like spinach, kale, and broccoli) into your diet. For more on eating right in pregnancy, see Chapter 1.

The cervix has heavy work to do in a multiple pregnancy. Even the simple act of standing has gravity working against you. In women with a short cervix (approximately 25 mm or less at 24 weeks), some reinforcements may be required. If cervical incompetence is suspected, a transvaginal ultrasound, in which the Doppler wand is inserted into the vagina rather than moved across the belly, is used to assess cervical length and monitor the progress of the cervix. As a preventative measure, your provider may suggest a cerclage—a procedure involving suturing (or stitching) the cervix closed to avoid preterm dilation. Studies are inconclusive as to whether or not cervical cerclage is effective in improving birth outcomes, but it does appear that the earlier cerclage is performed in the pregnancy, the more potential it has for success. Cerclage is usually performed in the second trimester.

Almost half of all multiple pregnancies result in preterm labor (labor before 37 weeks). If you start having contractions or other signs of preterm labor and are still less than 4 centimeters dilated, your provider may try to halt labor until you're further along in your pregnancy with one or more of the following methods:

- **Bed rest:** Strict bed rest may be imposed to keep the pressure off your cervix. This could be at home (with a few bathroom passes granted) or in a hospital. A fetal monitor may be used to keep an eye on the team's progress.
- **Fluids:** You may be hooked up to an intravenous line and/or fed fluids to keep you hydrated.
- **Trendelenburg position:** Bed rest—to the extreme. If your provider mentions this, he wants you on a bed that works against gravity by elevating your feet and tilting your head down.

- **Tocolytic medication:** Tocolytic drugs like magnesium sulfate, calcium channel blockers, and terbutaline may be administered by mouth or intravenously to stop contractions.
- **Antibiotics:** If your membranes have ruptured prematurely (preterm premature rupture of membranes, or PPROM), antibiotics can help to ward off infection. They are also used to prevent group B strep infection of the preterm newborn.

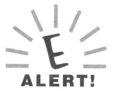

ALERT!

There are some situations where tocolysis should not be attempted, even if you are considerably preterm. If monitoring indicates that your fetus is in distress, if you have signs of infection of the amniotic fluid, if you are bleeding excessively, or if you are preeclamptic, tocolyctic drugs are not recommended. In most of these cases, immediate delivery by Caesarean section will be required.

If measures to prevent preterm delivery are unsuccessful, an amniocentesis can determine whether the fetal lungs are developed enough to breathe in the outside world (see Chapter 5 for more on amniocentesis). If results indicate that the lungs are still immature, injections of corticosteroids are administered to accelerate surfactant production while labor is held off as long as possible. The ACOG recommends steroid treatment for women expected to deliver at 32 weeks or earlier in pregnancy.

In amniocentesis of multiples, a blue dye is injected into each amniotic sac after a fluid sample is withdrawn. If the same sac is accidentally tested twice, the appearance of the dye will tip off the physician to the error. It's important that all sacs be tested whenever practical, since multiples often develop at different rates and may have achieved various levels of fetal lung maturity.

Problems Babies May Face

Up to 70 percent of monoamniotic twins and higher-order multiples experience umbilical cord knotting, twisting, or entanglement. In severe cases, kinks or tangles in the cord can cut off blood supply to one or both fetuses. Ultrasound can determine the presence or absence of a dividing membrane between multiples. If a multiple monoamniotic pregnancy is detected, it will be followed closely with routine ultrasounds to check for umbilical cord complications. Regular non-stress testing (NST) may also be employed to evaluate fetal health (for more on diagnostic tests, see Chapter 5).

Twin-to-twin transfusion syndrome (TTTS) is a rare condition affecting approximately 10 percent of those "identical" twins who share a chorionic membrane and placenta. In TTTS, an abnormality in the placenta causes irregularities in fetal blood circulation, and blood is shunted between the fetuses through placental vessels that connect them. The result is that one fetus experiences cardiovascular overload and potential heart failure, while the other receives insufficient blood flow. TTTS is not limited to twins and can occur in higher-order multiple pregnancies as well.

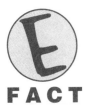

FACT

A laser-surgical technique developed in the 1980s can be used to successfully treat some cases of TTTS. Fetoscopic laser occlusion of the connecting placental blood vessels (FLOC) uses an endoscope (a thin, flexible tube with a tiny camera attached) to find the blood vessels connecting multiples and close them off.

In addition to its involvement with TTTS, the position and construction of the placenta can impact the growth of one or more multiples. Maternal blood flow and nutrition may be unequally distributed among fetuses, resulting in an uneven growth rate among them. Multiples are also at a higher risk for intrauterine growth retardation (IUGR). For more on that condition, see Chapter 13.

Vanishing twin syndrome is the death of one twin that was previously viable. When it occurs early in pregnancy, the body is typically reabsorbed into the uterine wall. Some minor bleeding and cramping may signal the process. More serious complications may result if vanishing twin syndrome happens later in pregnancy, including cerebral palsy in the surviving twin and potential circulatory problems in the mother.

Other conditions multiples are considered at high risk for include congenital abnormalities and placental problems (e.g., placenta previa, placental abruption). For more on these conditions, see Chapter 13.

Delivering Multiples

Nothing is routine in a multiples pregnancy, and the surprises will likely keep coming through labor and delivery as well. Close communication with both your health care provider and a neonatalogist (a physician who specializes in newborn and preemie care) about the possible scenarios you and your children face at birth will leave you better equipped to make informed decisions.

Caesarean versus Vaginal Delivery

About half of all twins are born via Caesarean section, and the number goes up considerably for triplets or more. Because of the risk of umbilical cord entanglement, multiples that share an amniotic sac are usually delivered by C-section at or before 34 weeks.

Whether other multiples are delivered vaginally or not will depend on how they are positioned in the womb. If the first baby is breech (feet or buttocks first), your provider will probably prefer C-section. If at least the first baby is vertex (head down), a vaginal delivery may be performed. Women who feel strongly about having a vaginal delivery of their multiples should speak with their provider early on in the pregnancy about the issue.

A quick ultrasound in the labor and delivery room will reveal your babies' positions. In some cases, external cephalic version may be attempted to turn a stubborn twin (for more on version, see Chapter 16). In most cases of twin vaginal birth, the provider will attempt to deliver the second baby within 15 minutes of the first to minimize possible complications.

Premature Birth

Babies who are born prematurely are at risk for respiratory distress syndrome (RDS) due to lung immaturity. According to the American Lung

Association, an estimated 60 percent of preemies born before 28 weeks experience RDS. After 28 weeks but before 34 weeks gestation, that figure drops to 30 percent.

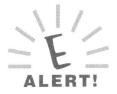

ALERT!

Preemies who develop RDS are also at risk for a lung disease called bronchopulmonary dysplasia (BPD). BPD occurs in up to 30 percent of infants who survive RDS and is triggered by trauma to the immature lungs from infection, respiratory therapy, or the stress of oxygen itself. Symptoms include wheezing, rapid breathing, cough, straining of abdominal and neck muscles, and a need for supplemental oxygen past 28 days of life.

Treatment for RDS may take several forms, depending on the severity of the condition. Animal-derived or synthetic surfactants may be administered shortly after birth to hasten lung maturation. An oxygen tube that fits under and into the nostrils may provide continuous positive airway pressure (CPAP) to force the alveoli (air sacs) of the lungs open. A newborn may also require intubation and breathing assistance with a mechanical respirator until lung function can develop further.

Postpartum Hemorrhage

Women who have delivered multiples are at an increased risk for postpartum hemorrhage, or excessive bleeding, after delivery. Some of the tocolyctic medications (e.g., magnesium sulfate) can also increase the risk of bleeding by inhibiting uterine muscle function. Once the placenta is delivered, the uterus must continue to contract in order to tamp down and seal off placental blood vessels. In a womb that is overstretched from multiples, the myometrium—the smooth muscle layer responsible for contractions—may not function efficiently. Postpartum hemorrhage can be the result.

If postpartum hemorrhage does occur, the uterus will be double-checked for any remaining pieces of the placenta (another cause of postpartum bleeding) and massaged to control the bleeding. Oxytocin or prostaglandin may also be administered to stimulate contractions.

When Babies Are in NICU

You've waited and waited to hold your babies in your arms, and now they're in the neonatal intensive care unit (NICU), behind glass and bound up by wires and tubes. Be assured that even though they may be dependent on machines, your presence and parental touch is critical in speeding their recovery and eventual discharge.

"Kangaroo care," skin-to-skin parental to preemie contact, has been shown to have a positive impact on parent-child bonding and improve the motor and cognitive development of premature babies. But early on, some very premature babies may not yet be ready for the sensory overload of touching. Be assured that they will want and need it as time goes on, and NICU staff and neonatal physical therapists can instruct you on methods of nurturing forms of touch for your children.

Never forget that your presence is essential to making this scary, sterile world a loving, temporary home for your children. Holding their tiny hands, getting involved with their care and feeding, and learning how to care for any unique medical needs are all critical tasks right now. The skilled nursing staff of the NICU can be a tremendous resource as you get comfortable with your children's care. Tap their expertise while you have the opportunity.

Barring any other serious medical problems, your new family members will be discharged from the hospital once they've reached a predetermined weight goal (usually around 2000 grams, or 4.4 pounds) and are able to maintain their body temperature and feed and breathe well on their own. If any of your children require special medical monitoring or attention after discharge, home visits from a nurse can help you get adjusted to their care routine. Turn to Chapter 13 for more on preterm birth.

Surviving the First Month Home

Be it hired help, grandparents, or friends, you absolutely must have backup support when you're bringing home multiples. Ideally, you'll organize your recruits well before birth, but this isn't always possible given the unpredictability of due dates with multiples. Think about designating a trusted friend or relative to delegate tasks—someone who's organized and dependable. Try not to stick your spouse with the job; both of you will have your hands full when the kids are finally here.

Schedules, Schedules, Schedules

Depending on the number of babies you're juggling and whether you're breast or bottle feeding, it may seem easier at first to just feed them all on demand. However, that strategy may eventually be at the expense of sleep and sanity. Without a little nudging, they will continue to follow their own timetable, the one that has you grabbing your shuteye in 20-minute stretches.

So how do you get your little ones with the program? A rigid feeding and sleep schedule is doomed to failure; newborns need to know you're there for them no matter what the agenda says. A more practical and flexible approach is to wake up all the babies once one awakens to eat. Feeding them all simultaneously and then laying them back down to sleep will get them on track toward a feeding schedule that's more or less in synch.

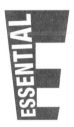

Your babies will probably not sleep longer than 2 hours at a stretch to start, so having them in your bedroom or getting a comfortable bedroll or inflatable mattress for the nursery floor may be a good idea for those nights that even finding your way back to bed seems too time intensive.

Breast, Bottle, or Both?

The moment you hear "multiples," breastfeeding takes on a whole new dimension. Visions of becoming a 24-hour, all-you-can-eat buffet for this litter of babies may have you revisiting your plans to nurse exclusively. Before you make any rash decisions, know that mothers of multiples can and do breastfeed (and live to tell about it!).

At the same time, don't let anyone tell you that it will be easy. It will take a lot of hard work and persistence—and an equal amount of support from family and friends—to nurse your babies successfully. But the health, bonding, and cost benefits can make breastfeeding multiples well worth your while.

Why breastfeed your brood? First of all, breast milk is cheaper and more convenient for a single baby; multiply that time and money savings by two or more and you end up with quite a deal. In addition, multiples may get an even bigger immunity boost from breast milk because of their tendency to be preterm and low birth weight babies, two factors that raise their risk for other health problems. And breast-feeding provides special one-on-one time with each child, a rare thing in "multiple-land."

Many moms of twins find that nursing both children at once (tandem nursing) is the most efficient way of taking care of feeding time. This may be a little tricky to master at the onset, but you'll get better with practice. An appointment with a lactation consultant is also a good idea for breastfeeding mothers of multiples to get pointers on scheduling, logistics, and more.

Football hold

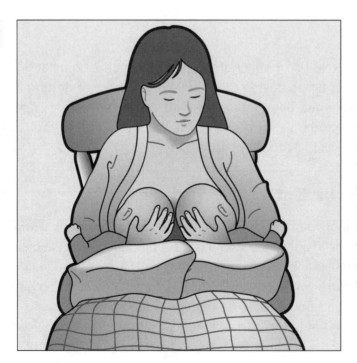

◀ Mothers of multiples can nurse two babies simultaneously in a number of positions—including the football, parallel, criss-cross, and front V holds.

Parallel hold

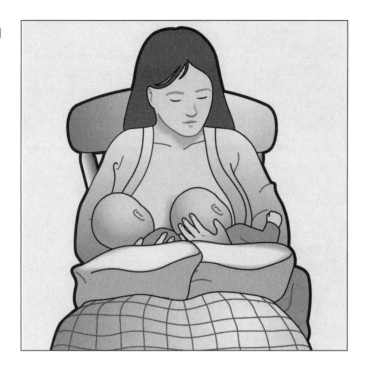

Criss-cross
hold

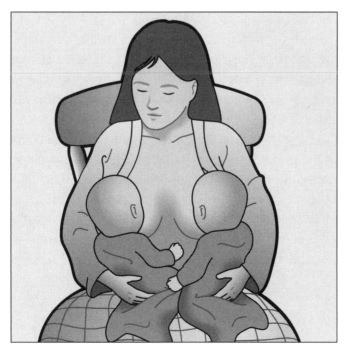

Front V hold

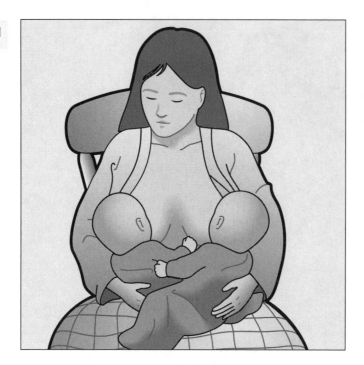

Bottle feeding can have its positives as well, particularly with higher-order multiples. The biggest benefit is that your husband or other helpers can get in on the action, a huge plus if you're trying to get two or more on the same feeding and sleeping schedule. And if you have an impatient eater in your crew, you don't have to worry about making him wait his turn while the others nurse.

Really want to provide your children with the health benefits of breast milk, but finding the physical toll of nursing multiples overwhelming? Some women choose to rotate a formula feeding among their multiples while the others feed at the breast. However, this may result in a diminished milk supply over time. Consider augmenting a few breastfeedings a day with a bottle filled with pumped milk instead. For more on breastfeeding, see Chapter 19. (E)

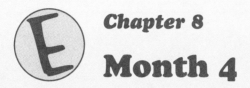

Chapter 8

Month 4

Welcome to the second trimester, or what many women consider "the fun part." Your energy is up, and your meals are staying down. You and your baby are headed into a period of rapid growth now, so hang on and enjoy the ride. Here's a look at what you can look forward to in month 4.

Baby This Month

Snoozing, stretching, swallowing, and even thumb-sucking, your fetus is busy this month as he tests out his new reflexes and abilities. He is losing his top-heavy look as his height starts to catch up to his head size. By the end of this month, he will measure about 6 to 8 inches in length and weigh approximately 6 ounces.

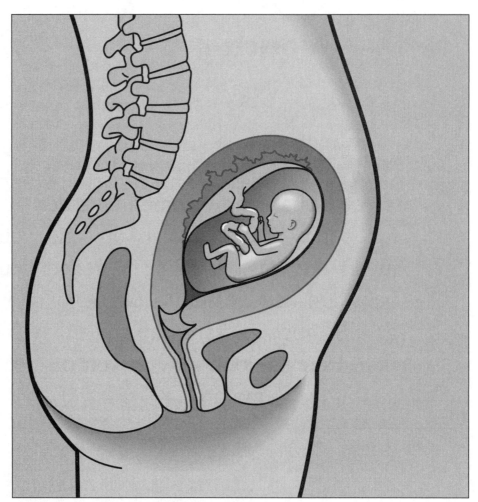

▲ You and your fetus in month 4 of pregnancy.

Now is a good time to begin singing, reading, and even playing music for your little one. The inner ear structures that allow him to hear are developing this month (for more on fetal hearing, see Chapter 12). He has grown eyebrows, eyelashes, and possibly even a little hair up on top.

The long bones of his arms and legs are growing as cartilage is replaced with spongy, woven soft bone in a process called ossification. Skeletal development will continue long after birth and well into adolescence and young adulthood.

Your baby is inhaling and exhaling amniotic fluid, practicing his technique for his first breath in the outside world. The lungs are already generating cellular fluid and a substance known as surfactant. In later months the surfactant will assist the development of the fetal lungs by expanding the alveoli, or air sacs, within them. These substances move out through the trachea and become part of the amniotic fluid, along with the urine your unborn child is already passing.

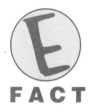

FACT

The umbilical cord contains two arteries and a vein sheathed with a gelatinous tissue known as Wharton's jelly. The jelly cushions the blood vessels and protects them from kinks and twists. Although umbilical cord knots do occur, they are relatively rare, happening in approximately 1 percent of pregnancies.

The placenta is approximately 3 inches in diameter this month, and the attached umbilical cord is about as long as the fetus and continues to grow. Fetal blood is being pumped through this little body at about 4 miles an hour, exiting through two large arteries in the umbilical cord and on to the placenta. In the placenta, baby's waste products (urine and carbon dioxide) are exchanged for oxygenated, nutrient-rich blood that is returned to the fetus via an umbilical cord vein. Pressure from the blood pumping within the cord helps straighten it out and keeps it from becoming knotted or getting in the way of your unborn baby's kicks and somersaults. Total time for this complex exchange? About 30 seconds.

Your Body This Month

In pregnancy, feeling is believing. While hearing baby's heartbeat or seeing fetal movement on an ultrasound monitor are milestone moments, the first time you actually sense your child inside of you—proof positive that you are indeed nurturing an actual human being—is a humbling and life-affirming experience.

Your Body Changes

If you weren't showing last month, chances are you will have a definite pregnant profile by the end of this month. Your uterus is about the size of a head of cabbage, and its top tip lies just below your belly button.

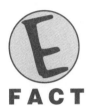

FACT

The thin line of fine hair that runs from your navel down to your pubic bone—the *linea alba*—may turn dark in pregnancy again thanks to hormonal changes. If you do develop this little stripe, now called a *linea nigra*, it will most likely lighten again postpartum.

What You Feel Like

Your appetite may start to pick up this month, especially if you've been too sick to enjoy a good meal until now. You'll need a healthy craving or two to fuel fetal growth—about 60 percent of your total pregnancy weight (about 11 to 15 pounds) will be gained in this trimester. (For more on weight gain in pregnancy, see Chapter 6.)

Heartburn may start to become a persistent problem as your uterus crowds your stomach and the smooth muscles of your digestive tract remain relaxed from the hormone progesterone. Some tips for putting out the fire:

- Avoid greasy, fatty, and spicy foods.
- Stay away from alcohol and caffeinated drinks (e.g., cola, tea, coffee); these may relax the valve between the stomach and the esophagus and exacerbate heartburn.
- Keep a food log to try to determine what your heartburn triggers are.
- Eat smaller, more frequent meals instead of three large ones.
- Drink plenty of water *between* meals to reduce stomach acid.
- Don't eat just before you go to bed or lay down to rest.

- Pile a few extra pillows on the bed to assist gravity in easing heartburn while you sleep.

If heartburn symptoms won't relent, there are several over-the-counter antacids and medications available that are considered safe to use in pregnancy. Speak with your doctor to find out which one may be right for you.

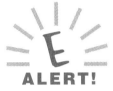
ALERT!

Calcium—it does a baby good. Your little one needs lots of calcium to build bone and blood cells, and if she doesn't get it in your diet, she'll draw on your skeletal storehouse instead. Milk is an excellent source; four 8-ounce glasses daily will provide you with the recommended 1,200 milligrams. Yogurt, broccoli, kale, and salmon are rich in calcium as well.

As if heartburn wasn't enough to deal with, pregnancy may start to become a real pain in the rear, literally. Many women develop hemorrhoids, which are caused by increased pressure on the rectal veins secondary to pregnancy. By straining to have a bowel movement, you put stress on the rectal veins, which can become blocked, trapping blood, turning itchy, painful, and perhaps even protruding from the anus. Exercise, a high-fiber diet, and plenty of water can help to avoid constipation and straining with bowel movements that may aggravate the condition. Try easing the pain with an ice pack, a soak in a warm tub, wipes with witch hazel pads, or a topical prescription cream as recommended by your doctor.

Hemorrhoids do have the potential to become more than just a minor discomfort, so be sure to speak with your provider about them if they do occur. While they typically resolve after pregnancy, in some cases clotting occurs, and surgery is necessary.

Other symptoms of second-trimester pregnancy you may start or continue to experience this month include:

- Nausea
- Fatigue

- Frequent urination
- Tender and/or swollen breasts
- Bleeding gums
- Excess mucus and saliva
- Increase in normal vaginal discharge
- Mild shortness of breath
- Lightheadedness or dizziness
- Gas and/or constipation
- Skin and hair changes
- Feeling warm or easily overheated

Movement!

Think that ultrasound was exciting? Just wait until you feel your little gymnast stretch and push inside of you for the first time. If this is your second or third child, you may already recognize the familiar sensation of her little body flexing in your slightly used womb. For moms in their debut pregnancy with somewhat less stretchy accommodations, the first movements—known as quickening—may not be felt quite as early. By week 19, most women have felt that distinctive first flutter.

So what does it feel like? It's often described in terms of butterfly wings or bubbles, or less poetically as gas or a block of jiggling Jello in the abdomen. Because pregnancy can cause so many gastrointestinal symptoms, you may not even notice the gentle nudges of baby until she's been persistent with her movements for a few days.

You'll quickly discover that your baby is already establishing behavioral patterns. When you're up and about, she may be rocked to sleep by your movements. It's when you lay down and try to take a rest that she wants to get up and groove. Is your partner having a tough time getting a hand on your stomach in time to feel the fetal kung fu? Have him stand by during a down time and see if he can catch a kick or two.

Once baby starts moving regularly, the sensation quickly becomes second nature. On average, you should feel four or more movements each hour from your passenger. Three or fewer movements or a sudden decrease in fetal activity could be a sign of fetal distress, so if you notice either call your provider as soon as possible to follow up.

The Shape You're In

Carrying high or low? Looking large or barely showing? It's practically inevitable that at some point in your pregnancy someone will guess the gender of your child based on how he or she is filling out your belly. While guessing is an entertaining way to pass the time, the theory that high means a girl and low means a boy has no basis in science. How you carry is dependent on your build, posture, and pregnancy history. Women who have had a previous pregnancy tend to have more pliable abdominal muscles and therefore often carry lower. The baby's position also influences your pregnant topography, which may change from one day to the next.

At the Doctor

If you didn't get a listen to the fetal heartbeat last month, you'll likely get your chance with this visit. Women who have chosen to take an alpha-fetoprotein (AFP) test will have their blood drawn sometime between week 16 and 18. For more on the AFP, see Chapter 5.

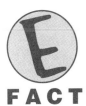

FACT

Varicella infection (chickenpox) can cause serious complications in pregnancy for both mother and developing child. If you have never had chickenpox and are exposed to anyone with chicken pox, contact your health care provider immediately. If your blood tests negative for antibodies to the virus, treatment with varicella-zoster immune globulin (VZIG) can be effective in preventing up to 80 percent of infection if administered early enough (within 96 hours).

On Your Mind

You're now hitting your stride as the wooziness and uncertainties of the first 3 months fade away, and the discomforts of late pregnancy still lie relatively far ahead.

Feeling better and having more energy, you may be ready to conquer the world (or at least the nursery). Yet coworkers, friends, and family now starting to recognize you as "a pregnant woman" may be handling you with kid gloves.

The pampering is nice, within limits. Accept the small favors that ease the discomforts of pregnancy—such as a closer parking space or the cushy chair in the conference room. But don't hesitate to be firm with those who try to pressure you to cut back on tasks you're perfectly capable of handling, or who treat you like a porcelain doll.

Reality Strikes

For many women, the starter's pistol on motherhood goes off right when they feel baby's first pokes and prods. The palpable presence of your child may trigger a series of mothering emotions—protectiveness, nurturing, nesting—and complete and total impatience with anyone who poses a potential threat to the well-being of you and your child.

This maternal defense system may seem a bit extreme to the husband who is banished from the bedroom when he has a head cold, or the visiting friend who is asked to take his cigarette outside in subzero weather, but you aren't being paranoid nor unreasonable. No one would think twice about keeping a newborn away from sneezing and smoking; a developing fetus is just as, if not more, vulnerable.

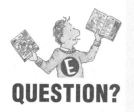

QUESTION?

Are my vivid dreams related to pregnancy?
Dreams that are exceptionally realistic, disturbing, or just plain bizarre are common in pregnancy. Your dreams are reflections of what's on your mind, so it's natural for them to reflect concerns about the baby, your family, and the future. They may seem larger than life right now due to insecurities about the future and again, those pregnancy hormones.

Exercise

Don't avoid the gym, pool, or other favorite fitness hangouts just because you're pregnant. Exercise will not only make you feel better, it can tone muscles that will be getting a workout in labor and delivery. Feeling alarmingly large among the gym babes? Try mixing up your routine with something new like hiking, golf (sans cart), or a prenatal exercise class.

So how much is too much? It depends upon your prepregnancy fitness level. If you were swimming 1 hour each day before pregnancy, there's no reason not to continue that routine if you have your provider's blessing. On the other hand, don't start training for a marathon if your notion of exercise is walking into McDonald's instead of using the drive-thru. The rule of thumb—for women in "regular" pregnancies (i.e., not high-risk), 30 minutes of moderate exercise daily is ideal.

Benefits

If you weren't into a regular fitness routine before pregnancy, exercise may be just about the least appealing thing you can imagine right now. Try to set your distaste aside for a few moments and consider the benefits a regular workout may provide:

- **Energy up.** Stretching and moving daily will boost your energy level and calm your mind.
- **Postpartum weight down.** It will be easier to work off your pregnancy weight after the birth if you already have a regular routine.
- **Ease your aches and pains.** Exercise that promotes strength and flexibility can prevent or diminish lower back pain, muscle aches, and other complaints of pregnancy.
- **Positive mental attitude.** Feeling fit may improve your self-image.

Staying Active

Exercise doesn't have to be complicated, expensive, or technically difficult. It can be as simple as tossing a ball with the kids in the back-yard, taking the dog on a brisk walk each evening, or swimming or even walking laps in the local pool. Again, 30 minutes of regular, heart-pumping activity started and capped off by a good stretching routine is all it takes to benefit you and baby. Above all, make sure it's an activity you enjoy or something done in good company so you will look forward to it.

If you thrive on routine and feel more likely to get moving if you have a set schedule, check out your local YMCA, hospital, or community center for a prenatal exercise class. Water exercise programs are also a good, low-impact way to get fit. Even if your class is tailored toward moms-to-be, check with your doctor first.

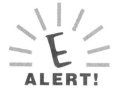

ALERT!

Certain activities are definitely off limits during pregnancy. These include scuba diving, water skiing, and contact sports. In addition, proceed with caution when participating in potentially high impact activities like tennis, volleyball, and aerobics. As always, run any new or prepregnancy fitness routine by your health care provider before you take part.

Precautions

While exercise can be a boon to your body and baby, there are basic steps you should take to stay safe. First and foremost, run your routine by your provider to get a medical stamp of approval. If you're new to working out, start slowly. Be attuned to your body's signals and stop immediately if you experience warning signs such as abdominal or chest pain, vaginal bleeding, dizziness, blurred vision, severe headache, or excessive shortness of breath.

Dress in supportive, yet comfortable clothing that breathes well and braces your belly and other parts of your expanding anatomy. If your feet have swollen past the comfort level of your old gym shoes, invest in a bigger pair. Drink plenty of caffeine-free fluids before, during, and after your workout to remain well hydrated, and try to work out in a climate-controlled environment to avoid an extreme rise in core body temperature, as overheating can be hazardous to a developing fetus.

Kegels are one exercise every pregnant woman should know and practice. They strengthen the pelvic muscles for delivery and can improve the urinary incontinence, or dribbling, some women experience in pregnancy. What's a Kegel? Tighten the muscles you use to shut off your urine flow, hold for 4 seconds, and relax. You've just done your first Kegel. Try to work up to 10 minutes of Kegels daily.

Just for Dads

Every couple bickers once in a while. In fact, many relationships seem to thrive on heated debate (think James Carville and Mary Matalin). But the hormonal tidal wave and stressors that accompany pregnancy may bring an unexpected degree of added friction to the mix. Try to remain sensitive to her physical and mental changes without being condescending. In other words, "Honey, I know it's just the hormones talking," is not a good way to resolve an argument.

Understanding Her Emotions

You can't feel her aches and pains, but you can feel the brunt of her volatile emotions.

Even if you understand why she's moody, with all this exposed emotional wiring, you may be tempted to keep a low profile. Remember, your partner needs empathy and assistance right now, not sympathy and avoidance. Support her with your actions, love, and acceptance, and you can make it through this pregnancy with an even stronger bond.

You may be starting to feel the "but what about me?" syndrome coming on. The hullabaloo surrounding your significant other and your unborn child may be making you feel a little (or maybe even a lot) neglected. Your partner is focusing on the pregnancy and baby instead of you, as well. Feeling left out, or even jealous, is perfectly normal. Try to address your feelings by arranging some special couple time for you and your partner where you both can be waited on and pampered a bit—splurge on a night out at a special restaurant, a weekend at a nice hotel, or a double massage. And also keep in mind that you have a very special role to play in this pregnancy too—as father-to-be, both mom and baby are relying on your support, coaching, patience, and love.

What You Can Do to Help

Be patient. You will be expected to use your mind-reading capabilities to their fullest extent. In other words, your partner may not ask for help, but you need to offer it (and offer it frequently). Then—and this is critical for the procrastinators among you—follow through soon after. If she is in nesting mode, chances are she won't let things sit undone for long. If you don't follow through, then all you've done is to compound her stress with irritation.

Volunteer for errands and chores that are starting to become physically difficult for her pregnant body, such as weekly trips to the laundromat, mowing the lawn, and taking your ill-behaved St. Bernard to the groomer. Let her sleep in on the weekends. Take care of some of those household repair tasks you've been meaning to get to before she has to remind you about them.

If you already have other children, it's easy to let your partner's rest and mental health needs take a back seat as other parental responsibilities come to the forefront. Consider getting some extra help around the house from relatives or even a biweekly cleaning service to keep things manageable. Don't miss Chapter 11 for tips on helping your family adjust to second or later pregnancies. (E)

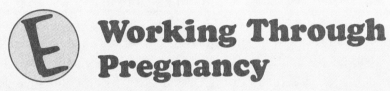

Chapter 9

Working Through Pregnancy

Worried about keeping up on the job during your pregnancy? Recognize your value, not just as an employee but also as a woman. Don't let anyone make you feel guilty about being pregnant. Know your rights, stick to your guns, and realize you don't have to settle for the status quo when it comes to the workplace.

Your Rights

Unfortunately, it's sometimes easier to change the legal employment landscape than alter prevalent workplace attitudes and prejudices. Too frequently, pregnancy is construed as a personal indication that you have no want or need for professional fulfillment.

Even if you do consider work nothing more than a way to pay the bills, your rights are still important. Intolerant and illegal attitudes toward pregnancy can result in financial loss as career advancement screeches to a halt, you get the minimum salary bump at your annual review, and bigger and better job offers dry up. Fortunately, federal and state statutes are in place to try to minimize the chance that you will be professionally or economically punished for your choice to become a mother.

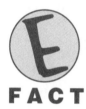

FACT

If you belong to a union, talk to your union representative about maternity and paternity leave under your contract. You may have additional rights and benefits that aren't available to nonunion employees at your workplace, and in some cases these may exceed the benefits covered by state and federal law.

The Pregnancy Discrimination Act

The Pregnancy Discrimination Act is a 1978 amendment to Title VII of the Civil Rights Act of 1964. The act requires that your employer provide you with the same rights, resources, accommodations, and benefits as other employees who are on temporary disability due to illness or injury. It also dictates that your employer must allow you to work as long as you are physically able to do your job. Keep in mind that the act only applies to businesses with more than 15 employees, and if your employer does *not* provide disability benefits to injured or ill employees, your comparable benefits will be just that—nothing.

If you're searching for a new position while pregnant, the Pregnancy Discrimination Act protects you from prejudice on the basis of your pregnancy. Still, legalities aside, pregnancy may make your interviewer look for other viable reasons not to hire you. It's illegal for a potential employer to ask if you're pregnant or not in the interview, and you certainly aren't required to volunteer the information. However, if the job is offered to you, it is probably in your best interest to mention your pregnancy during final negotiations. You want to start your working relationship off on the right foot and address any concerns your prospective employer has up front.

The Family and Medical Leave Act (FMLA)

If you or your spouse work for a public agency, a private or public elementary or secondary school, or a company with more than fifty employees for a period of at least a year, you have coverage under the Family Medical Leave Act (FMLA). The FMLA provides for up to 12 weeks of unpaid leave within a 12-month period for medical and family caretaking reasons, including the care of a newborn child. Both moms and dads are eligible as long as they meet the employment criteria.

The FMLA also enables you to take unpaid time off if you experience health problems during pregnancy and your employer does not provide disability or sick day benefits. The same goes for extended time off you might require to care for your child should she have any health problems at birth. Again, the total time off provided for under the FMLA is not to exceed a total of 12 weeks in 12 months.

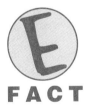

FACT

New parents who have been denied FMLA leave from their employer and believe they are eligible can file a complaint with the U.S. Department of Labor (DOL). The complaint must be filed within two years of the incident. Call the DOL at ☎1-866-4USWAGE for further information.

State Law

Depending on where you live, your state may mandate certain employee rights related to pregnancy and maternity benefits under Worker's Compensation laws. Check with the labor department or other applicable organization in your state to find out more.

Occupational Hazards

Depending on your position and work environment, you may have to alter your duties temporarily, or request a change in location or accommodations. If your job involves any of the following elements, talk with your human resources department about your options:

- **Weight lifting.** Lifting heavy packages, boxes, or other items is not recommended in pregnancy, especially past 20 weeks (e.g., shipping and receiving clerks, warehouse work).
- **Second-hand smoke.** Women who work in the hospitality industry (e.g., bartenders, waitresses) may expose their fetus to toxins in second-hand smoke.
- **High heat.** Excessive temperatures can be harmful to fetal development, particularly in the first trimester (e.g., summer construction, factory environment).
- **Teratogen exposure.** Jobs that involve working with certain chemicals and hazardous substances (e.g., welders and lead exposure) are linked to birth defects.
- **Standing and repetitive movement.** Line work or other jobs that keep you on your feet all day (e.g., factory jobs, assembly work, piece work) can exacerbate circulatory problems.
- **Ionizing radiation exposure.** Pregnant pilots and flight crew may be exposed to excessive ionizing radiation, another known teratogen. Radiographic imaging technicians that work with X-rays, CT scanning equipment, and nuclear medicine are also at risk.

Breaking the News

In an ideal world, the news of your impending motherhood would be greeted with congratulations and reassurance at the office. Instead, reality may find you strategizing against a negative employer reaction and determining the right time to drop the pregnancy bombshell for minimal fallout to your career. That pregnancy should be considered a handicap to be overcome rather than the positive, life-affirming force it is remains a glaring reminder of how far women still have to go to achieve equality in the workplace.

When you do inform your employer, make sure that they hear it from you, and not around the water cooler, first. Accompany the news with your tentative schedule for maternity leave so your manager can plan accordingly. Offering suggestions you have for a replacement in your absence or ways to temporarily reassign workload will reflect well on you and your perceived commitment to your employer. For more on "When (and What) to Tell Work," see Chapter 6.

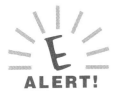

ALERT!

If you have a health problem in pregnancy you may find yourself facing an X-ray or similar exam. According to the American Academy of Family Physicians (AAFP), the maximum safe fetal radiation dose during pregnancy is 5 rad, or the equivalent of 50,000 dental X-rays or 250 mammograms. CT scans, fluoroscopic studies, and nuclear medicine tests involve slightly higher doses than conventional X-rays, but in general still fall well within the range of acceptable exposure. In each case, the benefits of imaging need to be weighed against the potential risk to the fetus, and if at all possible, tests involving radiation should be avoided in the first trimester of pregnancy.

Avoiding the "Mommy Track" Trap

Once you share your news, you may suddenly find yourself on a slow road to nowhere at work—last in the information loop and out of the running for promotions and job advancements you were previously an easy pick for. Goodbye fast track and hello mommy track?

Is it unavoidable? Not necessarily. Employers who realize that a happy employee is more likely to be a productive employee won't punish you for pursuing a personal life. And if you continue to perform well and make it clear to your supervisors and management that you'd like to have a career path with the company rather than just a job, you're more likely to avoid the so-called mommy track. Still, whether the mommy track exists in your organization or not depends on the corporate culture and the attitudes of upper management. Do they support family-friendly policies? Do they lead by example and use benefits like paternity leave themselves? And are efforts made to institute initiatives that benefit employees across the board, from the security staff to the CEO?

The Ideal versus the Real

In the real world, some organizations "reward" those who invest themselves more fully in the workplace than in family. The result is an atmosphere in which pregnancy is construed as a choice "against" company and career, one that may be tolerated for the sake of political correctness but certainly isn't supported through policies and rewards systems. The good news is that there are family-friendly employers who put their benefits packages where their mouth is. See where your company lies between these two extremes:

The ideal . . . a fully equipped lactation facility.
The real . . . a bathroom stall with a broken lock.

The ideal . . . paid time off for prenatal appointments.
The real . . . isn't that what lunch hours are for?

The ideal . . . expectant mother parking spaces near the entrance.
The real . . . unless you have an acronym after your name, it's first come, first served.

The ideal . . . a pregnant supervisor to commiserate with.
The real . . . your bachelor boss is a freshly minted MBA who thinks "family-friendly policy" means Christmas off with pay.

The ideal . . . a flexible schedule for your unpredictable pregnant body.
The real . . . don't forget to punch out for bathroom breaks.

The ideal . . . 4 months of maternity leave with full pay and benefits.
The real . . . with luck, that partial disability pay should arrive before your child's first birthday.

Defining Personal and Professional Goals

What do you want out of life, both personally and professionally, now that your family is changing? If this is your first child, it can be hard to fully assess the new direction you're taking. But there are probably some basic decisions you can make with a degree of certainty. For example, late shifts and double-overtime may be out of the picture for you now.

You may also have career goals that you'd like to keep on target. Should they be mutually exclusive of motherhood? No. May they be, depending on where you work? Yes. If you wanted to move into a supervisory position at your next review, but see your company promoting those who work excessive overtime, you have choices to make. Such is the delicate balance of motherhood. Fortunately, you always have the option to look for a workplace that is more in harmony with your personal and professional goals—or to take your own path, whatever it may be.

Realize Your Value

Think of full-time motherhood as another job offer on the table for your employer to stack up to. Your company may be willing to sweeten the pot with flex-time, telecommuting, or other family-friendly working arrangements to keep you happy. Remember, in most cases they have poured a significant amount of money and resources into your training. The loss of that investment, plus the cost of hiring and training a new employee, is a big financial incentive for keeping you on board. Don't be afraid to rock the boat. Realize your value and use it as a bargaining chip.

Negotiate Toward Your Goal

Think about using your maternity leave as a launchpad for alternate working arrangements. For example, if you would like more than the 6 weeks of paid leave your company offers and would ultimately like some flexibility in your schedule, suggest a work arrangement like telecommuting for the 6 weeks following paid leave. If you're covered by the FMLA, your employer must give you 12 weeks off without pay to care for your newborn if you request it. By offering an alternative to your complete absence, you appear flexible and dedicated, and your employer certainly has nothing to lose by trying it. Even if you aren't prepared to take 6 weeks off unpaid should your employer turn you down, it's well worth the gamble to suggest the idea. You can always scale back your plans if your request isn't granted. And if it is accepted and works out well, you will have proven yourself for a more permanent arrangement down the road.

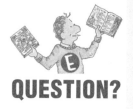

QUESTION?

I asked for 3 months of maternity leave and told my employer I'd work part-time for the last 6 weeks if the length of time were an issue. A week later they fired me, saying that I wasn't dedicated enough. What do I do now?
First, consider yourself lucky you discovered their un-family-friendly attitude now rather than later. Then, pick up the phone and contact your nearest U.S. Equal Employment Opportunity Commission office by calling ☎ 1-800-669-4000. If you're covered by the FMLA, your former employer has broken the law. Don't wait too long—the EEOC has time limits on when charges of employment discrimination can be filed.

Practical Matters

No matter what your job, staying comfortable, relatively stress-free, and economically secure during your pregnancy is essential.

Staying Comfortable

Women who work on their feet should make a habit of changing positions often and moving when possible. Wear comfortable shoes and consider support stockings.

For jobs that require a lot of sit-down time, make sure you have an ergonomically appropriate chair that promotes good posture. A lumbar support pad may also help ease pregnancy-related lower back pain, and you can put up your feet under your desk on a small stool or even a stack of phonebooks. If you work a desk job, look for opportunities to get up and about. Take a walk to speak with a coworker instead of picking up the phone or hand-deliver a memo instead of using interoffice mail.

Scheduling Doctor Visits

Hopefully, your employer recognizes that good prenatal care translates to a healthier, more productive employee and in the long run, less time spent out of the office to care for sick kids. However, if you do face resistance in taking time off for doctor's visits, remember that prenatal care is considered necessary medical care and is covered under the FMLA. If all else fails, you can invoke your legal rights.

In the meantime, find out if your provider has evening, weekend, or early morning appointments that might fit around your workday. If you must go during office hours and your supervisor isn't pleased, offer her the alternative option of taking the entire day of your appointment off as vacation or unpaid leave instead. Perhaps she'll look at your short absence in a new light.

If you're getting static for meeting basic prenatal care requirements now, just think what it will be like when you need time off to care for a sick child or keep a well-baby appointment. File a "family unfriendly" mental note for follow up post-pregnancy. Companies who score poorly in supporting their pregnant employees will probably continue the trend. If too many red flags are raised during your pregnancy, once you reach maternity leave it may be time to look for a company that realizes the value of both personal and professional fulfillment in their employees.

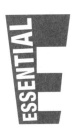

At the end of your rope with a real pain in the you-know-what? Write a no-holds-barred e-mail or letter to the PITA in question, but do not send it (leave his or her name off of it for now—nothing worse than hitting the send button by accident). Then let it sit overnight and revisit it the next day with a cooler and clearer head. Just airing your feelings will usually improve your outlook, and you can either edit it for tact and a PG rating or send it straight to the shredder or delete folder.

Controlling Stress

The workplace can be a stress hotbed. Deadlines, personality conflicts, difficult clients, quotas, overtime, and more make for a pressure cooker that's not good for you or baby. Try to maintain some perspective and peace of mind by realizing that petty office politics mean little in comparison to the health and well-being of your child. Turn to Chapter 4 for tips on coping effectively with stress.

Maternity Leave

Your bonding time with baby should be free of workplace concerns. If you plan appropriately for your departure and absence as early as possible, you'll get more out of your time off. It's a good idea to put all maternity leave plans in writing for your supervisor and appropriate managers, and to make an extra copy for placement in your personnel file.

Planning Ahead for Leave

Lay the groundwork for your maternity leave so there won't be too many questions or crises in your absence. If appropriate for your position, delegate some tasks to coworkers and arrange coverage by others. Find out if your supervisor plans on hiring temporary help to fill in during your absence, and work on training materials and checklists so you won't face a mess upon your return to the office.

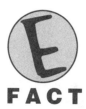

FACT

According to a 2001 benefits survey performed by the Society for Human Resource Management (SHRM), paid paternity leave was offered by 29 percent of midsized companies (2,501 to 5,000 employees), while only 13 percent of large companies (over 5,000 employees) offered the benefit. Even if your workplace doesn't offer paid paternity leave, dads may qualify for time off without pay under the Family Medical Leave Act (FMLA).

Check and double-check that all appropriate benefits paperwork has been filled out, signed off, and sent in well in advance of your planned departure. Maternity leave should be a low-stress time, not one that requires twice weekly contact with human resources to find out the status of your disability claim.

How Many Weeks?

So just how much, or how little, maternity leave should you take? Certainly the benefits your company provides will play a major factor in your decision. If you have quite a bit of seniority you may be able to swing an even longer leave by tapping into accrued vacation time. Other factors to consider include:

- **Money.** How much time off can you afford if your maternity benefits are minimal or nonexistent? Don't forget to factor any money you'll be saving (i.e., dry cleaning bills, lunches out, transportation expenses) into your equation.
- **Management.** Even though you may be legally within your rights, in some organizations an extended maternity leave may be frowned upon by those above you. Consider what management might think, and more importantly, what kind of priority you should place on their disapproval.
- **Morale.** Are your coworkers and/or subordinates happy and motivated, or disillusioned and bitter? Employees that work as a team and feel invested in their workplace are more likely to rise to the challenge in your absence.
- **Malleability.** Does it have to be all or nothing? Think about offering some creative proposals for extending your leave, such as a reduced part-time schedule or telecommuting.

Evaluating your leave options will reveal the pluses and negatives in your company's attitudes toward personal employee fulfillment. If morale is poor and management unyielding, once you've gotten past maternity leave it may be time to consider your options.

Back to Work

After you actually deliver your child, the toughest job you'll have is that first day back to work. You'll worry about whether his caregiver will be able to tell his hungry cry from his tired cry, if he's getting the attention he thrives on, and of course if he misses you. Try to focus on the benefits of the situation—the increased value of the time you do have together, his broadening horizons as he interacts with new children and adults, and the financial security your family is gaining.

Easing the Transition

No matter how you slice it, it's hard being away from your baby. If you can, start back on half days to ease into the separation. Drop in at day care during your lunch hour if it's logistically possible. Above all, make the most of the time you do have together by making home a work-free zone.

Striking a Balance

In your pre-mommy life, you may have set up certain expectations you find yourself hard pressed to live up to now. It's time to define appropriate work limits, even if it means pulling in old boundaries. Coworkers and clients who felt free to contact you before via pagers, wireless phones, or what have you, day or night, now need to be gently guided to keeping it to the office or at the least evaluating the urgency of their issues before picking up the phone. Getting some control back may be as simple as gradually ridding yourself of all the extra gadgetry that makes you painfully accessible and weaning your colleagues to voicemail or e-mail only access.

Women who work nontraditional schedules may have special needs for achieving balance. Evening "day care" can be tough to find without friends or relatives in the area, and scheduling that changes on a weekly basis can make child care even more difficult to plan on. Talk to your supervisor candidly about your needs and see if a shift change or a more permanent schedule can be arranged. If you're a dependable and valued employee, your employer would rather work with you to retain your skills and experience.

Changing Paths

A corporate culture that was perfect for your single lifestyle may just not fit your new family way of living. If the nature of your job or employer makes it impossible for you to achieve that delicate work/home balance, it may be time to change direction with a new employer.

Family-Friendly Companies: What to Look For

Few organizations will admit to being family *un*friendly when asked during the interview process. Uncovering the truth will take some detective work on your part.

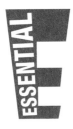

Finding out about flex-time options when you're still in the interview process can be a sticky situation. In many organizations, arrangements like telecommuting are still reserved as a privilege or reward (or even a necessary evil) for those who have proven their value to the company. Unless the job description includes flexible arrangements, you're better off not inquiring directly about the possibility. Instead, ask broad questions about available benefits and the "average" work day, which will reveal the information naturally.

You can look to resources like business-focused local and national media (both *Forbes* and *Working Mother* magazine put out an annual "100 Best Companies to Work For" list) as a starting point. Corporate annual reports can also be a good source of information. Once your foot is in the door and you're going through the interview process, make sure you have an opportunity to talk to potential coworkers and get an overview of available benefits and programs. A few programs and plans that may be a good indication a company is family friendly include:

- **Flexibility.** Does the company have written policies on options like flex-time, job-sharing, and telecommuting?
- **Lactation facilities.** Are there appropriate, comfortable areas dedicated to breastfeeding or breast milk pumping? If not, is your

employer willing to provide an appropriate, private space?

- **Paid paternity leave.** Are dads given time off for a new baby with pay, or at least without prejudice? If a policy is in place, is it used successfully?
- **Onsite child care or child care assistance.** If your workplace doesn't have onsite or sponsored child care, does it offer enrollment in a tax-free flexible spending account that allows you to save up to $5,000 tax-free to pay child care expenses?
- **Time-saving perks.** These may run the gamut from onsite dry cleaning and retail services to employee concierge services that can run small errands for you.
- **Value placed on education.** Corporate-sponsored scholarships for children of employees, tuition assistance, and mentorship programs with local schools are a few ways a company may express the value of education.

Flex-time, Telecommuting, and Other Options

Even if your company doesn't have established flexible working options, it can't hurt to pitch the idea to your supervisor or to the human resources department. There's always a first, and you may be blazing the trail for others who will follow you.

First of all, realize that your position needs to be conducive to the arrangement you're suggesting. If you have a computer-intensive desk job that could be performed remotely with a simple dial-up connection, you're more likely to get a telecommuting arrangement than a receptionist, whose job description requires her physical presence. Look at what type of flexible arrangement your position might mesh with. For example, job sharing might be perfect for the receptionist and a coworker.

Create a proposal that is well researched and realistic. Outline just what you want out of the arrangements, in specific terms including hours and logistical requirements (such as home computer equipment). Cover your contingencies, such as the ability to be available for onsite meetings, even if you aren't scheduled to be at the office.

Make sure you outline the potential benefits to your employer as well. For example, if office space is at a premium in your building, a telecommuting arrangement will free up your desk for other employees. If your employer has no track record of flexible scheduling programs, the resulting boost in employee morale and company image is also a plus for their reputation.

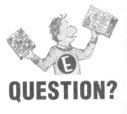

QUESTION?

I want to keep breastfeeding, but my company doesn't have lactation facilities. Any suggestions?
As more and more companies are seeing the value in family-friendly policies, perks like lactation lounges are becoming more commonplace. Talk to your human resources department about possible options at your workplace. Sometimes an unused storage area or empty office can be at least a temporary solution. If all else fails, you may be able to arrange something with a sympathetic coworker who has an office (with a door that locks so the copier repairman doesn't wander in). The bathroom is a last resort option, but it's exceedingly difficult to get your milk to let down while you're balancing a pump and associated apparatus in a bathroom stall. You'll also find that a pump can be *loud*, and the acoustics in bathrooms are good, which can add to the awkwardness.

Finally, the fact that you're making the suggestion reveals that you might consider greener pastures without accommodations to your needs. If that happens, your employer loses time, talent, and money—the three things corporate America wants to grow, not squander. Make it easy for them to say yes by putting together a well-considered and realistic proposal.

Full-Time at Home

Becoming a full-time mom is an exciting new venture for many women. If you can afford to stay home without working for someone else, go for it. Pouring your skills and knowledge into parenthood can be enormously fulfilling, and in fact is probably the most rewarding job you'll ever have.

Finally, for the woman who wants it all and wants it close to home, consider the possibility of forging your own family-friendly path. In today's wired world, many occupations lend themselves to home-based work—writing, income tax preparation, desktop publishing, and Web design are naturals. If the field you currently work in is unfulfilling and you'd like to make a change, look to the hobbies you enjoy for some ideas. Refinishing antiques, creating crafts for retail, sewing, and painting are a few that might be a good fit for a new career. Starting something new is never easy, but sometimes just looking at the miracle of your child helps you see the possibilities.

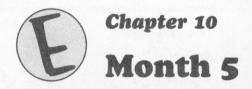

Chapter 10

Month 5

Y ou're still enjoying the relative comfort level of the second trimester, but your energy and initiative may be slightly dampened by the dwindling quality of your sleep. Sleep deprivation can also contribute to mental fuzziness and emotional edginess. If you haven't already, start to value and prioritize time spent between the sheets (asleep, that is).

Baby This Month

At 10 to 12 inches long and around 1 pound in weight, your baby is about the size of a regulation NFL football. How appropriate, considering you've reached the half-time of pregnancy.

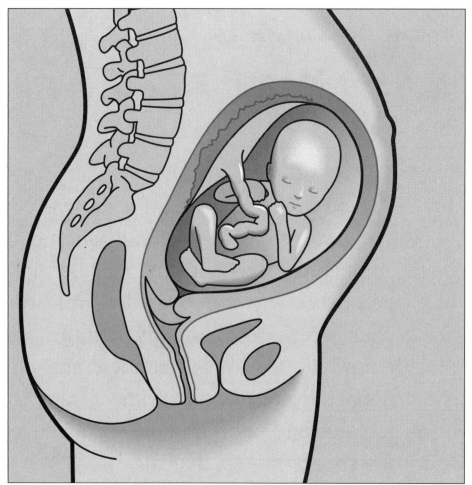

▲ You and your baby halfway to the end zone.

Your little linebacker is starting to bulk up a bit as she accumulates deposits of brown fat under her skin. This insulation will help regulate her body temperature in the outside world. She's using her bulk to make her presence known; if you weren't feeling her last month you likely are now. A look at her through ultrasound might reveal a wave of her clenched hands, which open and close freely now and have their own unique fingerprints.

The fetus is now covered in a white oily substance known as *vernix caseosa*, a sort of full-body fetal Chapstick that keeps her fluid-soaked skin from peeling and protects against infection. Some of the vernix will remain on the baby at birth, particularly in the skin folds (more if she is early, less if she is post-term).

Your Body This Month

As baby grows, your muscles and ligaments stretch to support this new weight. The result may be a new set of aches and pains as your body adjusts to the load.

Your Body Changes

Feeling like you're turning inside out? Your "innie" may have already become an "outtie" as the skin of your belly (and accompanying button) is stretching, tightening, and itching like crazy. A good moisturizing cream can relieve the itching and keep your skin hydrated, although it won't prevent or eliminate *striae gravidarum*, or stretch marks. Whether or not you'll develop stretch marks is largely a matter of genetics, although factors such as excessive weight gain and multiple gestations may increase your odds of having them.

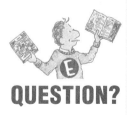

QUESTION?

I was expecting stretch marks, but not varicose veins! What's up with that?
The hair-fine marks, also known as spider veins, usually appear on the lower legs and are caused when increased blood volume and pressure damage the valves that regulate blood flow up out of the blood vessels of the legs. The result is pooled blood in the vein and that telltale squiggly red or blue line. Supportive stockings, putting up your feet, resting on your left side, and taking an occasional walk when you need to stand for long periods of time may relieve leg soreness associated with varicose veins.

The red, purple, or whitish lines of striae are created by the excess collagen your body produces in response to rapid stretching of the skin. They may appear on your abdomen, breasts, or any other blossoming body part right now. Don't be too alarmed, as striae typically fade to virtually invisible silver lines after pregnancy. If you do feel self-conscious, there are some options for postpartum treatment of severe cases (see Chapter 21).

What You Feel Like

The band of ligaments supporting your uterus is carrying an increasingly heavy load. You may start to feel occasional discomfort in your lower abdomen, inner thighs, and hips called round ligament pain. Pelvic tilt exercises are useful for keeping pelvic muscles toned and relieving pain.

The pelvic tilt can be performed while standing against a wall, but may be most comfortable done four-on-the-floor style. Keep your head aligned with your spine, pull in your abdomen, tighten your buttocks, and tilt your pelvis forward. Your back will naturally arch up. Hold the position for 3 seconds, then relax. Remember to keep your back straight in this neutral position. Repeat the tilt three to five times, eventually working up to 10 repetitions.

The root of all things uncomfortable—pregnancy hormones—are also contributing to lower back pain you may be experiencing. Progesterone and relaxin—the hormone responsible for softening your pelvic ligaments for delivery—are also loosening up your lower back ligaments and disks, and combined with the weight of your growing belly your back is feeling the strain. Women who are having twins or more are especially prone to lower back pain, which occurs in up to 50 percent of all pregnant women.

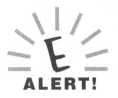

If your abdominal and/or back pains are severe or accompanied by fever, vomiting, vaginal bleeding, or leg numbness, call your health care provider immediately. Most minor back pain of pregnancy is completely normal, but in severe cases it can also be a sign of preterm labor, kidney infection, or other medical problems.

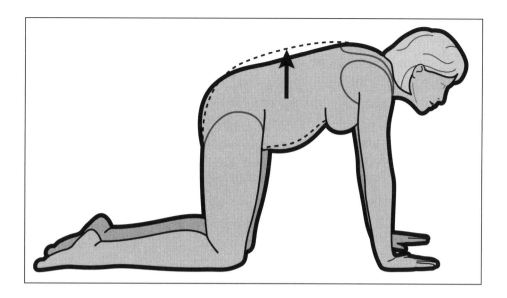

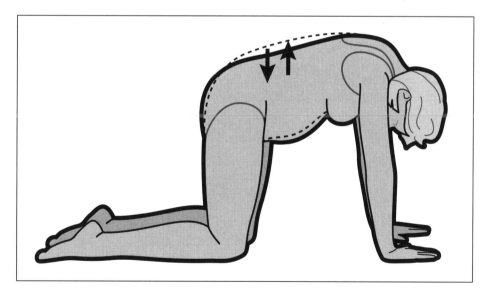

▲ Pelvic tilts can tone your perineum and ease pregnancy aches and pains.

A few tips to help you ease your aches and pains:

- **Stand tall.** Perfect posture can go a long way toward easing back pain. Try to keep your center of gravity in your spine and pelvis rather than out in your belly, which can give you a swayback.
- **Sit up straight.** Use good posture when you're sitting as well, and choose a chair with good lower back support. You can also purchase a special ergonomic support pad for your chair back, but a small pillow may do the trick just as easily.
- **Avoid twists and turns.** With everything so loose, a sudden move as simple as quickly turning at the waist to get out of bed may strain your back. Use your arms as support for a slow take-off when rising from a chair.
- **Practice your pickups.** If you have small children that still need to be lifted occasionally, it's essential to use good form. To avoid injury, bend and use your leg muscles to lift things rather than bending from the waist and lifting with your back.
- **Warm up.** A warm pad on your back, hips, or other sore spots may help relieve pain.
- **Sensible shoes.** Avoid high heels! They will place further stress on your spine, and they're anything but comfy these days.
- **Foot rest.** Use a low stool or step to rest your feet when sitting. If you must stand for long periods, alternate resting each foot on a step.
- **Massage.** You now have a medical excuse to indulge in a regular back rub from your significant other. A licensed massage therapist who is experienced in prenatal massage may also be helpful.
- **Fluff and stuff.** Sleep on your side with a pillow placed between your legs. This will align your spine and improve your sleeping posture. A full-sized body pillow or beanbag may help support your back and belly as well.
- **Exercise.** If you aren't doing them already, some stretching and flexibility exercises may be in order. Check with your health care provider for approval and recommendations; if the pain is troublesome enough or if you have a history of back problems, she may suggest a physical therapist to work with.

Feeling hot and bothered, and not in the fun sense? Pregnancy-induced changes in your metabolism and added weight may have you cranking the AC. Dress comfortably, cool off in the shower or tub, and invest in an extra fan if you don't have air conditioning.

Other symptoms you may start or continue to experience this month include:

- Nausea
- Fatigue
- Frequent urination
- Tender and/or swollen breasts
- Bleeding gums
- Excess mucus and saliva

- Increase in normal vaginal discharge
- Mild shortness of breath
- Lightheadedness or dizziness
- Headaches
- Gas, heartburn, and/or constipation
- Skin and hair changes

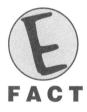

FACT

If round ligament pain is an increasing problem, you may consider buying a belly support band or belt, available at many maternity and baby supply stores. These bands cradle your growing abdomen and may ease your ligament and lower back pain. Check with your provider to see if one might be a good fit for you.

At the Doctor

Beyond the usual weigh and measure routine, your doctor may administer a glucose tolerance test (GTT) at the end of the month (between weeks 24 and 28). If she hasn't discussed counting fetal movements before, she may mention it now.

Now that you're halfway through pregnancy, you may be thinking more about labor and delivery issues. It's never too early to ask your doctor questions about what's on your mind. It's also a good time to start gathering information on childbirth classes from your local hospital or birthing center. There are several different methods of childbirth education, such as Lamaze, Bradley, and Bing; researching them now will give you and your partner time to learn more about which one is right for you. Even if you have experience in the delivery room, you can still benefit from a refresher course. Register early, but try to pick a class date that falls in your third trimester so the information will still be fresh in your mind once the big day arrives. Chapter 14 details some of your education options.

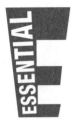

Having a planned C-section? You'll still benefit from prepared childbirth classes, which typically offer a comprehensive look at the entire birth experience, including hospital policies and procedures, newborn care, and a sneak peek at the maternity ward and nursery. Mention your caesarean when you call for information; some programs offer special classes just for moms who are having C-sections.

On Your Mind

There's bound to be an uncomfortable episode or two while your emotions are so close to the surface. Couple this emotional tension with your ever-growing list of things to do, and meltdown is imminent. Try to defuse the situation ahead of time by having an action plan for coping with anger-provoking situations.

Irritability

Because of all the added demands on your body, mind, and emotional balance, you may be finding yourself short on patience these days. In pregnancy, the proverbial molehill quickly becomes the mountain. You have absolutely no tolerance for the idiosyncrasies of others, and people you found mildly annoying before pregnancy may become absolutely impossible to be around.

If you can't stand your coworker's endless prattle about who did what to whom and got away with it, tell her you need some quiet time. And the next time your neighbor launches into her 303 easy steps for making your home look as great as hers, politely excuse yourself for a rest rather than letting your boiling point rise. Pregnancy is the perfect excuse for steering clear of people who—let's face it—are just plain annoying. Of course, avoidance isn't the ultimate answer, but during this crucial time where your emotional and physical balance are so important, it's a good solution for taking care of the little things and keeping your sanity intact.

If family and friends are getting your ire up as well, it may be a sign that you are feeling overwhelmed and undersupported. Take a look at what's really getting to you. When you blow up at your partner for forgetting to stop at the dry cleaners, is it because you really had to have your winter sweaters back posthaste or is it because lately you feel like you have to either nag or do it yourself to accomplish anything? If it's the latter, sit down and tell your partner what you're feeling, and work out some strategies for easing the burden together.

Overwhelmed

Half of your pregnancy has passed you by, and the baby's room is a sea of boxes, you can't decide on a name, and your office isn't even close to being ready for your maternity leave. Step back and take stock. Are you making work, and stress, for yourself through self-imposed deadlines? Look at your "to-do" list in terms of small tasks rather than an all-or-nothing prospect. Prioritize what's there and dare to cross off a few things that just aren't that important right now. It's nice to have everything *just so* for baby's arrival, but your new son or daughter is only going to care about three things—being warm, well-fed, and near her mom and dad.

Also remember that you aren't in this alone. If you're single, enlist family or close friends to help out. And if you are married but still aren't getting the help and support you need from your husband or family, ask for it. Although it's nice when others anticipate your needs and pitch in voluntarily, they may be wrapped up in their own preparations and anxieties about the new family addition. Don't feel guilty about reminding them that their help is needed now.

Sleeping Tight

Perhaps it's nature's way of preparing you for the sleepless nights to come, but your growing belly and the pushes and prods of your little one are making it increasingly difficult to get the requisite 8 or more hours of peaceful slumber. Sleep is essential to your mental and physical fitness right now, not to mention that of your child. Make your best effort to rest often and rest well.

Making Time

You work a full day at the office, go to the grocery store, come home and make dinner, stay up late working on the baby's room, and next thing you know it's midnight. Sleep is a priority right now, one you need to make time for. Make a regular bedtime, and stick to it. Leave major cleaning, errands, and home projects for weekends or other days you are off work or have extra help. If hitting the hay late is unavoidable, try to make up your sleep deficit with a weekend nap.

Getting Comfortable

The fetal sleep cycle is only between 20 and 80 minutes long, so if you aren't a sound sleeper you may find yourself awakened by baby's stretching limbs. Getting comfy may be a challenge if you were a dedicated stomach or back sleeper prepregnancy. Lying on your back puts undue pressure on your inferior vena cava, the vein that shuttles blood from your lower extremities (feet and legs) to your heart, and can trigger a drop in blood pressure. It's also extremely uncomfortable for any length of time by now. Logistically and medically, the best position for sleep right now is on your side.

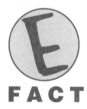

FACT

Left side sleeping enhances blood flow exchange with the fetus. Why is the left side preferred? Because the liver resides on your right side, and sleeping on that side positions your heavy uterus right atop it. That said, right side sleeping won't really hurt anything in a typical pregnancy, so if you wake up on your right, don't panic.

Hip and shoulder pain may be another source of sleepless nights, and one that's difficult to avoid since you must sleep on your side. If you've tried the tips for aches and pains outlined above and the pain is still keeping you awake, experiment with a foam egg crate cushion on your mattress for a little added padding.

You don't know what living is until you've had the luxury of stretching out full (and pregnant) on an acre of crisp cool sheets. If you don't have one already, and it's in the budget, contemplate upgrading to a king-size bed. The extra room will enable you to bring a body pillow or beanbag into bed to support your stomach and ease your back. Your partner will benefit, too, as he'll be less likely to waken at every toss and turn.

Another bedroom habit you may have picked up in pregnancy is snoring. Many women are mortified, and self-conscious, about this new development. After all, there's nothing that makes you feel more attractive than the thunderous vibration of your own nasal passages, unless it's waking up with a trail of dried drool on your face! The snoring may be related to a number of factors, including pregnancy-related nasal congestion, your increased need for oxygen, swollen airway tissues, and compression of the muscles that control breathing. Most of the miracle remedies and devices you see on TV will do little but cost you money. Your snoring will likely fade away after pregnancy. For now, invest in extra earplugs for your mate instead.

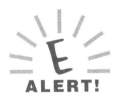

ALERT!

If you have been experiencing regular, sleep-disturbing snoring, make a point of mentioning it to your doctor or midwife. In a 1999 study, Swedish researchers linked chronic snoring in pregnancy to high blood pressure, edema (swelling), and low birth weight. They also found that habitual snorers were more likely to experience preeclampsia than infrequent or nonsnorers. If you snored excessively prepregnancy, you could have a sleep disorder known as sleep apnea that should be assessed by a doctor.

Make sure your environment is as sleep-friendly as possible. The room temperature should be cool enough for your overheated metabolism; your partner may want to stock up on extra blankets to get him through these occasional chilly nights. If ambient noise is a problem, get some earplugs or a white noise conditioner to cut the clamor. Keep a nightlight plugged into your room or hallway to navigate those inevitable late-night bathroom breaks with minimal injuries.

More tips for preparing yourself for a good night's sleep:

- To avoid heartburn, don't eat immediately before bunking down, and have an extra pillow on hand to elevate your head.
- Make the bathroom the last stop before bed.
- Stock your nightstand with crackers if you still wake with an unsettled stomach.
- If tender breasts are keeping you awake, wear a jogging or other supportive bra to bed.
- Stay away from caffeine (it isn't the best thing for you right now anyway).
- Don't exercise up to 3 hours before bedtime.

Just for Dads

Although your partner is still in the relative calm and comfort of the second trimester, you may be bone tired, as her tossing, turning, and expanding territorial stake of the bed has you sleeping fitfully. Some earplugs, or perhaps even an occasional night on the couch or guestroom bed to recoup sleep losses, can be invaluable. You may also be thinking more, perhaps with some apprehension, about your impending dad duties. Instead of worrying, take action.

Practice Makes Perfect

It's often said that a new baby doesn't come with an owner's manual or instruction book, but that's not completely true. Most hospitals and birthing centers will offer you a small forest of literature on how to care for your child once you get him home. Between this, prenatal education classes, and the hundreds of baby books at your local library and bookstore, you can at least gain an understanding of how all the parts are supposed to work.

However, if you're feeling a little insecure about your capabilities, getting some hands-on experience with a living, breathing baby can be a real plus. Offer to take care of a niece, nephew, or neighbor's child so you and your partner can get some baby care practice (Hint: don't use the word "practice" when offering babysitting services to their parents). If you're not quite up to the flying solo skill level yet, the next time you're visiting take the opportunity to hold, feed, or (if you're feeling daring) change the baby. Your interest will be welcomed; parents love an extra set of hands.

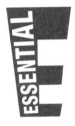

According to the National Sleep Foundation, up to 15 percent of women experience restless leg syndrome, or RLS, in late pregnancy. Characterized by pain or unpleasant sensations in the legs that are only relieved by movement, the exact cause of RLS in pregnancy is not known. It may be related to nerve compression or an insufficient intake of folate and/or iron. If RLS is keeping you awake, talk to your health care provider about treatment options.

The Second Time Around

Perhaps you're an expert at all of this dad stuff already, and you've been coasting through this pregnancy with ease. You still have some unknowns to deal with, including how your existing child or children are going to handle the mantle of siblinghood. Don't forget that every pregnancy is different, and what could have been smooth sailing last time may be tougher this go around (or vice versa).

Also keep in mind that even though you don't have new dad anxieties to contend with, your partner still has to do the heavy work. Share child care duties, take time to pamper her, and make her feel like a supermodel mom-to-be rather than the old lady that lives in the shoe. For more on second or later pregnancies, see Chapter 11.

Chapter 11

Repeat Performance: Second or Subsequent Pregnancies

Maybe you've been around the block before and consider yourself an expert at this pregnancy stuff. Even if the physical side of pregnancy is familiar, the emotional and mental aspects involved with each new child are always different. Families change with each new member. Yours will be no exception.

Baby and Your Body

Women who have been through pregnancy already (known as *multigravida* in clinical lingo) have some definite body benefits when it comes to carrying and delivering their baby. On average, labor is typically shorter, and these women are statistically less likely to need an episiotomy.

In addition, you'll probably feel your little one stirring earlier than your first, primarily because you can identify the sensation this time. Depending on the tone of your abdominal muscles, which may be laxer after your first pregnancy, you may also start to show earlier.

Every Pregnancy Is Different . . . Or the Same

In pregnancy, practice doesn't always make perfect. Just when you think you have it down, Mother Nature may throw you a curveball. You may have been horribly nauseous throughout your first pregnancy, and not even have a gas bubble this time around. Or, your second pregnancy may be filled with all sorts of strange, new symptoms. It's also possible that your second pregnancy may be a carbon copy of your first. Each baby has its own genetic blueprint, its own site of implantation, and its own unique placenta. The environment and life circumstances each child is born into may be vastly different as well. On the other hand, all of your pregnancies share the same maternal infrastructure, which may account for similarities in labor and delivery, pregnancy complications, and so forth. So will this pregnancy be the same or different? You'll just have to wait and see.

VBAC or Another C-section?

"Once caesarean, always caesarean" is an out-of-date obstetrical concept. Although many factors are involved in the decision to repeat a C-section (e.g., high-risk pregnancy, fetal position, type of incision made in the first section, scarring of uterus, number of previous C-sections), many women *can and do* try vaginal birth after caesarean (commonly known as VBAC). According to the ACOG, the success rate of VBAC is between 60 and 80 percent.

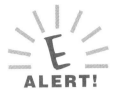

ALERT!

In the days before a transverse (or horizontal) caesarean incision was the obstetrical norm, VBACs were often discouraged because of the risk of uterine rupture. Rupture might occur when a weakened scar from a first C-section burst open under the pressure of strong contractions. Clinical studies have shown that prostaglandins can increase the chance of uterine rupture in VBAC, and the ACOG does not recommend their use in labor induction of VBAC for this reason. The use of oxytocin in a VBAC labor should also be closely monitored. (For more on labor induction, see Chapter 18.)

In women who are considered appropriate candidates for VBAC, vaginal delivery is often encouraged over C-section because of the potential complications involved with surgery (e.g., infection, hemorrhage). If you are having a VBAC, your provider may prefer that you deliver in a hospital equipped to handle a C-section if one becomes necessary. The ACOG recommends this type of setting, but many midwives don't believe this is necessary in an uncomplicated pregnancy scheduled to deliver by VBAC. Again, this is highly dependent on your medical history. If you are considered to be at low risk, a birthing center or even a home birth may be a reasonable choice for you. Consult your provider for her take on the situation.

If you had a difficult labor and delivery that ended in C-section with your first child, and you really want an elective (or planned) C-section this time, discuss the option with your provider. It will benefit you to find out the pros and cons on VBAC so your decision is a fully informed one, but in the end, it should be up to you.

Do keep in mind that another C-section will also require a longer recovery period than vaginal birth, something to consider when you already have children that must be cared for postpartum in addition to your new baby duties. However, recovery may seem a bit faster than getting back on your feet after your first C-section just because you've been through the process once and know what to expect.

Sharing the News

Don't be too disappointed if your news isn't met with the fanfare your first pregnancy announcement was greeted with. People tend to be a bit more laid back in reacting to second or subsequent pregnancies, which actually may be a better approach in helping your children adjust to the news.

With an Only Child

Telling your other child or children may not be all you had imagined it would be either. The reactions you get may run the gamut from happiness to horror. But involving the kids in the pregnancy from the beginning can benefit you all in the end. Even the child who has been begging for a little sister or brother will have some adjustments to deal with. If you know the gender of the new baby, it may have some bearing on how your child takes the news as well. Girls and boys who envisioned a resident same-sex playmate may be crestfallen when their plans are detoured. Friends with siblings may give your child an earful on how boys, and girls, operate. Don't worry—your little one will eventually come around.

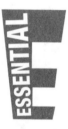

If you have a toddler or preschooler, consider waiting until the first trimester draws to a close to clue them in. Your due date might as well be in 10 years considering how slowly time seems to pass from a young child's perspective. Adding this short delay may make the wait more bearable. Of course, there is no one-size-fits-all. Consider your child's unique temperament in deciding when to share the news.

Should you reveal the gender if you know it? You know your child, and her personality, best. For example, if she doesn't like surprises and takes a while to warm up to new situations, you may want to let her know so she can prepare herself (particularly if she's making grand plans for her sister and a brother is coming).

If you have the opportunity, exposing your child to a friend or relative's baby may pique her interest in just how these little people work. Children who have absolutely no interest in sharing you may be coaxed into a more optimistic attitude if you're able to involve them in the pregnancy.

With an Older Sibling

Older children can be involved with your pregnancy much earlier and will probably enjoy helping you consider new baby names, hearing the baby's heartbeat, seeing their sibling on the ultrasound screen, and other milestone events of pregnancy. If they're old enough and have expressed an interest in helping out with baby care once their brother or sister arrives, you might even sign them up for a babysitting course through your local Red Cross.

In Blended Families

Blending families and stepsiblings at any age can be a challenge. Giving your children or stepchildren time to make a healthy adjustment to their new family unit prior to a pregnancy is probably the best way to set the stage for a new sibling. Even if your family is relatively young, all of you (especially stepsiblings) may be brought closer together by this new common bond in your family life.

Still, along with the uncertainties any child experiences about a new baby in the family, a stepsibling may question his place in the new family unit even more. Will the new baby replace him or her in your mind? Will she receive the lion's share of love and attention because both her parents live in the household? Involving the kids throughout the pregnancy, stressing their importance as siblings, and being supportive when they struggle with the transition are the best ways to ensure your family comes through pregnancy stronger than ever.

On Your Child's Mind

Getting comfortable with the idea of having a sibling, sharing parents, and potentially sharing a whole lot more will take a little time. Don't rush your child, or expect instant excitement at the idea of a new baby. Each kid adjusts in his own way, on his own schedule.

Keeping your child's life relatively consistent on other fronts can help him or her adapt to the new baby better. Now is probably not the time to start a potty training push, a move to a new house, or a change of day care providers. Stay on an even keel so she doesn't get overloaded.

Of course, some transitions, such as starting school, may not be avoidable. If a change is to occur, make sure it is cast in a positive light and its significance is duly noted, even if your household is in pre-baby chaos. The first day of kindergarten is a big deal, and should be treated as such.

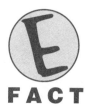

FACT

Some household changes, like moving your child into a big-kid bed so the new baby can have his crib, may seem small to you but may make your child uneasy and even resentful. If he has to move into a new room before baby's arrival, give him the chance to plan and decorate it. Even the youngest kids can have some input on the decorative scheme (e.g., Barney versus Pooh Bear motif).

Fetus Rivalry

Even before birth, your unborn child is taking a lot of your time and attention, especially in your other kids' eyes. Turning home life into a baby-centric universe where every discussion involves their sibling's arrival is a surefire way to get their guard up and may even make them question their importance in the family. Of course, talking about the baby's arrival is inevitable and healthy, in moderation. Just make sure the discussions don't exclude your other children.

If pregnancy is making you experience symptoms like nausea and vomiting that have you running slower than usual, your child may blame his sibling-to-be for your condition: "Mom can't go to the beach *again*. That baby is causing trouble already, and the little pipsqueak isn't even born yet!"

Assure your child that the way you are feeling is "normal" and is not caused by their brother or sister directly, but is instead just a part of pregnancy. You might even relate stories of your pregnancy with him or her if it was also plagued by morning sickness or other discomforts.

What's Happening to Mom?

Younger children are generally clueless about how a baby comes into the world. Stories of baby-dropping birds and kids popping out of cabbage patches may have them thoroughly confused. A good age-appropriate children's book on the subject can help you communicate the mechanics of the miracle of pregnancy and birth if you find yourself at a loss for words. Heidi Murkoff's *What to Expect When Mommy's Having a Baby* (HarperFestival, 2000) is an excellent choice for preschoolers and early elementary kids. Your local children's librarian should also be able to point you in the right direction.

When talking about conception, pregnancy, and birth with your child, there are a few things you need to remember:

- **Be straightforward.** Don't fall back on the stork. Age will make a difference in how much your child wants or needs to know, but when you do answer questions, try to call a penis a penis, not a ding-ding, tinkler, or other adorable euphemism (as tempting as it may be). Giving your child the right words to explain what is happening to your body and his family is a way to empower him and demystify this sometimes scary process.

- **Minimize the minutiae.** At the same time, don't take them from fallopian tube through baby's head crowning. Not only will they be bored spitless, but they'll probably tune out shortly after sperm meets egg.

- **Answer all queries.** As pregnancy progresses and becomes more visible and therefore more real to your child, questions may start to form in his mind. How can the baby breathe? How will she come out? What's she doing in there? Open the door for communication and ask your child occasionally if she is wondering about anything.

- **Make it relevant.** Kids love to hear stories about their own infancy and "fetal life." Pull out the baby book and home movies, and explain what life was like when they were the new arrival.

- **Explain the emotion.** Don't forget to let your child know why you've chosen to bring another family member into the fold. Let her be aware of the intense love surrounding the choice to conceive and to bring her a sibling she can love as well.

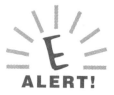

ALERT!

Once it becomes clear that a new baby is on the way, you may notice some behavior regressions in your younger child. Wanting to use a bottle, having potty training accidents, and other "baby" behavior is her way of saying she still needs you. Don't get angry with your child for slipping back into old habits, but do reinforce positive behaviors and point out the pluses and privileges of acting like a "big kid" (e.g., if you talk like a big kid instead of using baby talk, you can learn how to answer the telephone).

Needing Reassurance

Even the most well-adjusted, confident kid will need reassurance once in a while that he's still the apple of your eye. Don't let your world revolve around baby preparations so much that it overshadows special time spent with your other children. And make sure you give your child or children every opportunity to be involved with your family expansion so they can feel needed and wanted.

Involving the Sibling(s)-to-Be

Making your child a part of the pregnancy process is imperative to starting siblinghood off on a positive note. A kid who is relegated to the sidelines while everyone is focused first on your pregnancy and then on the baby is going to resent this new intruder, with good reason. Start the getting acquainted process before birth, and let your child talk and sing to her little sister or brother, help decorate the new baby's digs, and take on other important tasks.

Sibling Classes

Many hospitals offer classes for new siblings as a companion to their roster of childbirth education programs. When done right, an "official" preparation—complete with nursery tour, baby (doll) practice, and in some cases a diploma—can make even the most reluctant big brother or sister feel special and important in his or her new sibling's eyes.

Sibling classes can also give your child a chance to air his fears among peers and receive reassurance that he isn't alone in worrying about this squalling, needy creature that's moving in soon. Discussions about how other households are handling baby preparation, sleeping arrangements, and mom's upcoming trip to the hospital can also address concerns that your child hasn't thought of or hasn't felt comfortable verbalizing.

Classes should be small enough for discussion and interaction with peers and the instructor, and should ideally be separated into appropriate age groups. See Chapter 14 for more on sibling classes.

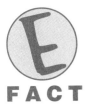

FACT

A good way to start the sibling relationship off on a positive note is to pick out a special gift from the new baby to his big brother or sister, and present it during their first meeting. Your new addition will be receiving copious amounts of attention, praise, and gifts, so this little gesture may symbolize a lot to your other child.

Through the Ages

Preteens and adolescents might be more receptive to the idea of a new sibling, simply because they're entering a phase in their development where they are focusing less on you and more on friendships and their social circle. A 14- or 15-year-old doesn't "need" you in the way a toddler, preschooler, or elementary school child does. You've gone from "mommy" to "mom" in their eyes, and a baby doesn't pose the same threat for your affections.

The Second-Time Father

Dads often feel that they have a bigger role to play in a second or later pregnancy, as the lion's share of child care often falls to them while mom deals with pregnancy symptoms. This is a great opportunity for you to spend time doing things with your kids that your spouse normally gets to handle, and to help them adjust to baby's upcoming arrival.

Of course, all this together time can have its pitfalls, too. While you may find yourself appreciating your wife even more when you have to take on tasks that she seems to handle effortlessly on a daily basis, that awe may sour to resentment as you realize that things won't change back to the old way anytime soon. If you feel overburdened, ignoring the problem is not the solution. Stress is bad for both of you, but particularly for the growing baby that's the focus of all these changes. Don't let it get the best of your family.

Get help from nearby family members, or hire sitters and household help if necessary. Even a neighborhood high school student can be useful to your spouse as a mother's helper. And remember that your older kids may be ready and willing to take on new responsibilities in the family. The key is to communicate how you're feeling, without blame, and work on a way to resolve the problem together.

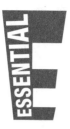

Don't forget that your significant other also has more to cope with this time around. It may be harder to find the time to offer some pampering when you have kids who need your attention, but be creative and try to do what you can to ease the burden. If she has primary responsibility for day-to-day child care, giving her a little time to herself—even if it's just enough for an evening walk or a 15-minute adult conversation with a close friend—is really essential.

Living Large: When You Choose a Big Family

One is wonderful, two is terrific, three—well you're starting to lose me but I guess I see the benefits. Four? Are you NUTS? If you have chosen to have a big family, you are probably used to this kind of reaction. Or perhaps you're just getting into the sizeable stage now, and haven't learned to shrug off the "when are you moving into the shoe?" comments yet.

The U.S. Census reports that in 2000, the lifetime average number of children for women nearing the end of their childbearing years was 1.9.

That's well below the average of 3.0 that was reported in 1980, and less than the 2.1 births per woman required for the natural replacement of the population.

Whether your reasons are religious, rooted in your own upbringing, or simply spring from a desire to have a home bursting with life and love, the bottom line is—it's your choice and your family. Don't let others make you feel freakish, or worse yet, like you're neglecting the children you already have, just because you choose to have more than the national average. A child is one of the greatest gifts you can give your family and community.

The success of a family lies in parenting quality, not in offspring quantity (big or small). Ignore the naysayers and remember that there are pitfalls and positives to every family configuration. There are enough theories and studies on sibling personality traits and birth order psychology to fill a not-so-small library. Although fascinating to read, trying to base your future family structure on them is next to impossible. Not every middle child will be the easy-going mediator of the family, and not every only child will be a hopeless perfectionist. Instead, use the lessons in them to avoid possible parenting pitfalls.

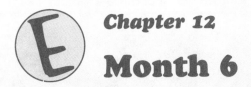

Chapter 12

Month 6

At month 6, you may feel as though you'll be pregnant forever, but the final trimester will come and go before you know it. Take some time this month to savor pregnancy, warts and all, and treat yourself to some of the indulgences that only a mother-to-be can pull off.

Baby This Month

Feeling a rhythmic lurch in your abdomen? Your little guy probably has the hiccups, a common phenomenon thought to be brought on by drinking and/or breathing amniotic fluid. They'll go away on their own, eventually; in the meantime, enjoy your little drummer boy and take advantage of the beat to let your partner feel the baby move.

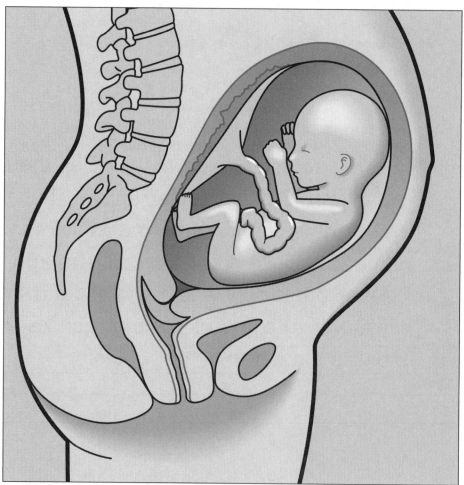

▲ You and your baby at the 6-month mark.

The once-transparent skin of your fetus is starting to thicken, and sweat glands are developing below the skin surface. He's over a foot long now, and by the end of the month may weigh up to 2 pounds.

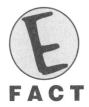

FACT

You hold more than your child within your uterus; you also are accommodating the origins of your grandchildren. If you're having a girl, your fetus has already developed an estimated seven million eggs in her ovaries by 24 weeks gestation. The eggs will be enveloped in small sacs called follicles as pregnancy continues, and by birth the number of eggs will have decreased to around a million.

He may now startle (or react) to a loud noise or other stimulation. Because his auditory system (the cochlea and pathways in the CNS) has developed enough to sense and even discriminate among sounds readily, he is becoming accustomed to your voice and others who talk "to" him frequently. Studies have demonstrated that newborns show a clear preference for their mother's voice, and for songs they heard while in the womb. Now is a good time to brush up on your lullaby repertoire.

Some clinical studies have found an association between exposure to excessive noise during pregnancy and high-frequency hearing loss in newborns. And while you can wear earplugs, your baby doesn't have the luxury. To stay on the safe side, you may want to avoid concerts, clubs, and other high-volume environments now. If your job involves heavy noise exposure, talk with your doctor about possible risks.

Your Body This Month

Your uterus extends well above your navel now. You may actually be seeing fetal movement across your abdomen as baby gets comfortable in his shrinking living space. As baby seems to get more nimble, you feel exceedingly klutzy—breaking everything that isn't nailed down, tripping over your own swollen feet, and taking out low-lying knick-knacks with your burgeoning belly. Blame it on your shifting center of gravity, and be careful if you're walking in slippery or icy conditions.

Your Body Changes

If the shoe fits . . . consider yourself lucky. Few women are able to fit into all their prepregnancy shoes for 9 whole months. What's behind all the swelling? The dramatic increase in blood volume you've experienced in order to nurture your child is feeding excess fluids to surrounding tissues, resulting in edema (or water retention). To make matters worse, the weight of your uterus is requiring the veins in your legs to work double time to pump all that extra blood back to the heart. And, of course, another culprit is (say it together everyone)—pregnancy hormones, as estrogen increases the amount of fluid your tissues absorb.

The result of all this is puffy and sometimes aching feet. Putting your feet up when you can, wearing comfortable low-heeled shoes, and soaking your feet in cool water are all good ways to ease the discomfort. Special compression stockings, available at medical supply stores, may also be helpful.

Don't restrict fluids or sodium—although avoiding excess sodium intake is fine, you actually need slightly more sodium in your diet in pregnancy to maintain your electrolyte balance. Fluids are crucial as well to prevent dehydration and keep you and baby well.

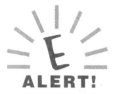

ALERT!

If you experience sudden and severe swelling of the face and hands, call your doctor immediately. It may be a sign of preeclampsia, or toxemia, a condition that is potentially hazardous to both you and your baby. Other signs of preeclampsia include high blood pressure, headaches, visual disturbances, sudden excessive weight gain, and protein in the urine. To learn more about preeclampsia, see Chapter 13.

What You Feel Like

You may have added leg cramps to your laundry list of pregnancy complaints. Stretching out your calf muscles can often quash a cramp, so the next time one hits extend your legs and point your toes toward your head. Some providers may suggest calcium supplements to ease cramping, but clinical studies are inconclusive as to whether or not this treatment is effective (although it can't hurt, given your increased calcium needs right now). A number of studies have found, however, that oral magnesium supplementation can be useful in alleviating cramps in some women. Check with your health care provider to see what she suggests.

Leg cramps can also be triggered by compression of your sciatic nerve—a condition commonly known as sciatica. Sciatica can also cause numbness and burning pain down the length of your leg and in your lower back and buttocks. Try stretching, a warm compress, or a tub soak for relief. And if you haven't already, review the tips for dealing with lower back pain in Chapter 10. If sciatica becomes more than a minor annoyance, talk to your health care provider. A date with a physical therapist may be in order.

If your leg pain is accompanied by swelling, redness, and skin that is warm to the touch, call your health care provider to report your symptoms. You may be experiencing deep vein thrombosis (DVT), a blood clot in your leg that impedes circulation and has the potential to embolize, or break off and block a major blood vessel. Pregnant women are five times more likely to develop DVT than their nonpregnant peers due to a slow-down of blood flow and an increase in clotting factors. However, DVT itself is relatively rare, occurring in less than 1 of every 1,000 pregnancies. If DVT is diagnosed, intravenous anticoagulant drugs are typically prescribed to treat the clot, and bed rest may be advised.

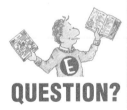

QUESTION?

Can the seat belt in my car hurt the baby? Should I stop wearing a shoulder belt?

Definitely continue to buckle up throughout your pregnancy. The lap belt should fit snugly under your belly bulge, and the shoulder belt should be positioned between your breasts. Don't worry about the belt hurting the baby; the uterus and fluid-filled amniotic sac are excellent shock absorbers. It's much more dangerous to you and your child to go beltless and risk being thrown from the car or into the dashboard in an accident.

Other symptoms on the menu yet again this month include:

- Nausea
- Fatigue
- Frequent urination
- Tender and/or swollen breasts

- Bleeding gums
- Excess mucus and saliva
- Increase in normal vaginal discharge
- Mild shortness of breath
- Lightheadedness or dizziness
- Headaches
- Forgetfulness
- Gas, heartburn, and/or constipation
- Skin and hair changes
- Round ligament pain or soreness
- Lower back aches
- Mild swelling of legs, feet, and hands

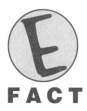

FACT

According to the 2000 U.S. Census, 6 out of every 10 American women between the ages of 15 and 44 are mothers. Kentucky led the nation in highest state rate of moms, with 67 percent of women holding the honor (compared to a 57 percent national average).

At the Doctor

More of the same this month as your provider checks your weight and fundal height, listens to baby's heartbeat, and finds out about any new pregnancy symptoms you may be experiencing. If you're reporting swelling, your provider may check your feet and hands. And, of course, no prenatal visit is complete without a urine sample and blood pressure check.

If you weren't given a glucose tolerance test to screen for gestational diabetes last month, it will probably be administered now.

On Your Mind

Now that your belly is too big to *not* notice, it becomes somewhat of a conversation piece. At first, you may be surprised to find women you don't know asking about your due date or the gender of your baby. The next question will inevitably be, "Is this your first?" Welcome to the sisterhood of motherhood.

The "What If" Game

Every new mom-to-be spends some time worrying about the health of her unborn child, especially if she's in a high-risk pregnancy. Take comfort in the fact that you've almost made it to the third trimester and your chances of delivering a healthy and happy baby are increasing each and every day. Obsessing over what could go wrong rather than focusing on living well will accomplish nothing but stress, insomnia, and anxiety—three things that are bad for you and baby. If you haven't already, turn to Chapter 4 for more information on stress management, and read on for some stress-busting techniques to release your worries and relieve your mind.

Enjoying Your Pregnancy

As you sidle up to the third trimester starting line, try to take advantage of these final days of relative comfort and sit back and savor—yes, *savor*—your pregnancy.

Pamper Yourself

Splurge for a day spa treatment. Spend a lazy afternoon curled up with a good book. Cool off with a dish of your favorite Ben & Jerry's flavor while you enjoy a nice relaxing soak in the tub. Take a scenic weekend drive with no deadlines or particular destination. Pampering yourself can relieve pregnancy symptoms, give you (alone or with your partner) special time to reflect on your future, and recharge you for what lies ahead.

Make sure you treat yourself to the little conveniences right now, too. Use the valet service to park instead of hiking from the lot, or shop at stores with expectant mother parking front and center. Too tired to cook at the end of the day? Order healthy carry-out fare from your favorite restaurant. If it's only lunchtime and you're already beat, arrange for an offsite play date for the kids for a few hours and have a midafternoon snooze. It may feel decadent at first, but taking the easy way out is a good thing right now.

Don't Stress

It bears repeating—again—that getting stressed out these days just isn't worth it for you or your growing child. Of course pampering yourself is one good way to lighten the load. But some women find they just can't enjoy a good old-fashioned self-indulgence day because they're too busy worrying about all the things they should be doing instead. If you fall into this category, don't add to your burden through forced relaxation that will only leave you tense and perhaps out several hundred dollars to boot.

Instead, use that money to whittle down your "to-do" list. Hire a cleaning service, send out the laundry, pay someone to do that painting in the baby's room, have the groceries delivered instead of schlepping to the supermarket. If your financial resources are limited, let your loved ones know you could really use their help right now, and don't be shy about delegating tasks when assistance is offered.

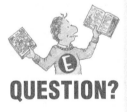

QUESTION?

Is it safe to eat or drink Nutrasweet while I'm pregnant?
Nutrasweet is the trade name for the sugar substitute aspartame. The FDA has determined that the sweetener is safe for most people to consume. To be safe, limit diet drinks to one a day. However, if you are pregnant and are diagnosed with hyperphenylalanine (high levels of the amino acid phenylalanine—a component of aspartame—in your bloodstream), you should stop using the product immediately, as excessive levels of this amino acid can cause brain damage. People with the genetic disease phenylketonuria (PKU) or advanced liver disease should also avoid aspartame.

Spending Time with Siblings-to-Be

Watching your child marvel at the changes in your body while he considers the possibilities of a new little sister or brother can be one of the most fun and fulfilling parts of pregnancy. Yet even the most enthusiastic sibling-to-be has some doubts about how he will fit into the new family unit. Unfortunately, those insecurities may only be intensified as you spend more time in the coming months visiting the doctor, going to childbirth classes, and tying down loose ends before the big day. Make sure you and your child or children have an opportunity each day to play, read, or just talk. You'll both benefit from this special time together.

Couple Time

With you in the pregnancy limelight and all the attention your agile, rib-thumping fetus demands, you may have inadvertently started to think of you and the baby as a couple. Your husband or partner is not an orbiting moon, although he may feel like one from time to time. Make sure he knows that he plays a valuable role in this pregnancy, and take the time to reconnect with him emotionally and physically.

If these are your final few months as a childless couple, take advantage of your freedom and spend some time doing your favorite grown-up things, activities that don't involve visiting the doctor's office or shopping for cribs and strollers.

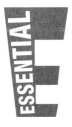

If you're both still ready, willing, and up to the challenge, sex can be more fun than ever. You don't have to worry about birth control, and the creativity required to find a comfortable position may inspire you to new heights. If the two of you are so inclined, oral sex may be a good option; just make sure your partner is aware that he should not blow into your vagina due to the rare but real risk of an air embolism. Women in high-risk pregnancies should consult their doctor about the safety of intercourse right now.

Just for Dads

Pregnancy is a special, one-of-a-kind time in your life as well as your partner's. From "My boys can swim!" to "Breathe, honey, breathe!" this long, strange trip will bring elation, anxiety, anticipation, and much more.

It will also give you the opportunity to see your partner in a whole new light: to watch her grow physically and personally as she makes the amazing transformation to motherhood. Her strength and sheer stamina in this 9-month marathon may have you feeling both proud and protective.

A Brand New Lifestyle

Yes, life will change significantly once your child arrives. No running out to catch a late movie and dinner at your favorite Mexican spot. You've got Disney matinees and Happy Meals on your dance card. Barney and his smiling minions will eventually muscle out your Monty Python video collection for shelf space. Going to work out will mean a trip to Gymboree or the local tot lot. But the first time your daughter smiles at you, or says your name, or laughs out loud at jokes that no one else would, it will all be so very worth it. And before you know it, you'll actually start to enjoy this second edition of your childhood from the parenting perspective.

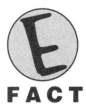

FACT

Planning on taking her out for a nice romantic dinner? Some advance planning will make the evening more enjoyable. If you can, pick a restaurant that is completely smoke-free; even designated nonsmoking areas can smell of lingering cigarette smoke if ventilation is poor. Make reservations so she won't be waiting on her feet for too long, and request a booth if one is available to give her more room to spread out. With her sometimes-fickle stomach, now is probably not the time to get adventurous with new cuisines, so stick to something tried and true.

Dads Should Enjoy Pregnancy Too

Unfortunately, even though we're well past the pacing waiting-room dads of the 1950s, fathers often get shut out of the pregnancy experience. The result can be frustration and anxiety. Many fathers-to-be experience significant stress related to the upcoming pressures of parenthood, but everyone's focus on mom and baby can minimize your concerns and leaves you feeling excluded.

It isn't just a matter of the "What about me?" syndrome. Dads who do try to connect with the pregnancy on a deeper level are sometimes ridiculed for their efforts. Ever get laughed at when you tell others "'we're' pregnant"? Or perhaps you're the type who snickers when the other guy announces his pregnancy (come on, you know who you are). Either way, you may end up internalizing your questions and fears due to a misguided sense of stoicism and consequently distancing yourself from the pregnancy experience.

Obviously, you'll never be able to fully experience pregnancy in a physical sense (nor will you probably want to after watching the woman you love live through it), but you can increase your emotional investment in this pregnancy by communicating with your spouse or partner about your hopes, dreams, and anxieties. Feeling stressed about your ability to parent, or about how your relationship with your partner may change, or about the possible upcoming financial changes in your family is completely normal. Talking about these issues as a couple can bring you closer together and help alleviate your worries. And the next time someone scoffs at "your" pregnancy, you might remind him that without your boys, there would be no baby. Ⓔ

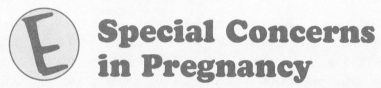

Chapter 13

Special Concerns in Pregnancy

Health problems, both those that pre-date your pregnancy and worrisome symptoms and conditions that pop up during the gestation, can be difficult to deal with. Staying educated and informed can reduce related stress and will help you take the best care of both baby and your body.

Chronic Illness and High-Risk Pregnancies

If you have a chronic illness, such as type 1 diabetes, you'll probably be referred to a perinatologist for obstetrical care if there's one in your area. Make sure your primary care specialist remains an integral part of your health care team throughout your pregnancy. Any changes to your treatment should be made in consultation with your doctor, and likewise any significant changes your specialist makes in your treatment during your pregnancy should be brought before your perinatologist. Open communication during this critical time is absolutely essential; if any of your providers aren't willing to be team players, find someone who is.

You will be making more frequent visits to all your health care providers throughout pregnancy to ensure that your illness remains well controlled and is not adversely affecting your unborn child. Any conditions that may potentially be transmitted to your child (e.g., HIV, herpes) either in the womb or during delivery may require drug therapy and/or potential caesarean section as well.

If you have concerns about your child inheriting your condition, a trip to a genetic counselor can be extremely helpful.

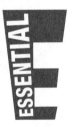

Your baby's development is mapped by the 46 chromosomes inherited from his or her parents (23 from mom and 23 from dad). Genetic blood testing of the parents can reveal if they are "carriers" of certain hereditary conditions that may be passed on to their child. Testing of fetal DNA through amniocentesis or CVS can diagnosis a chromosomal abnormality while the fetus is still in the uterus.

Genetic Testing/Counseling

Couples who are considered at risk for certain pregnancy problems due to age, ethnicity, family history, history of repeated miscarriage, or exposure to teratogens may be referred to a genetic counselor for a risk assessment. You may be given the option for further genetic testing—

which may include alpha-fetoprotein (AFP), amniocentesis, chorionic villus sampling (CVS), or level-two ultrasound—and provided with detailed information on the conditions in question.

Hereditary and chromosomal conditions that genetic testing can reveal include, but are not limited to:

- Down Syndrome
- Trisomies (three copies of a chromosome instead of two)
- Tay-Sachs disease
- Sickle cell anemia
- Cystic fibrosis

Genetic testing can also reveal certain birth defects. For more details on what to expect from a visit with a genetic counselor, see Chapter 1.

Ectopic Pregnancy

Ectopic pregnancy occurs when implantation takes place outside of the endometrial lining. In the majority of cases, it occurs in the fallopian tube, which is why it is often referred to as a tubal pregnancy. However, an ectopic pregnancy may also implant in the ovary, cervix, abdominal cavity, or cornual portion of the uterus (close to the fallopian tubes).

Unfortunately, pregnancy implantation must occur in the endometrium of the uterus for a pregnancy to safely continue. Allowing a pregnancy to progress in the fallopian tube or other ectopic site will result in tubal or other rupture in the first trimester, unavoidable fetal death, and potential maternal death. If you are diagnosed with an ectopic pregnancy, it will need to be surgically removed or treated with the drug methotrexate. Early treatment can preserve your fertility for subsequent pregnancies.

Women who have had previous ectopic pregnancies, who become pregnant with an IUD contraceptive device in place, who have a history of endometriosis and/or pelvic inflammatory disease (PID), and who have had a tubal ligation procedure are at a higher risk for ectopic pregnancy. The March of Dimes estimates that one in fifty pregnancies are ectopic.

Early signs of ectopic pregnancy include low hCG levels (hCG should approximately double every 2 days in a normal pregnancy), irregular bleeding, and pain. An abdominal or transvaginal ultrasound can usually confirm the diagnosis. If it remains undiagnosed, ectopic pregnancy is potentially life-threatening and can endanger future fertility. Warning signs that an undetected ectopic pregnancy may have ruptured include:

- Severe abdominal and/or pelvic pain
- Vaginal bleeding
- Dizziness
- Shoulder pain
- Nausea and vomiting

If you experience any of these symptoms, seek medical care immediately.

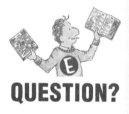

QUESTION?

Our ultrasound detected choroid plexus cysts in our baby's brain—what does that mean?
If no other abnormalities were seen on the scan, these small cysts that appear on the choroid of the brain have an excellent chance of resolving themselves by around 24 weeks with no ill effects to your child. The cysts are of note because in a small number of cases they have been associated with the serious chromosomal abnormality trisomy 18 (Edwards syndrome). Ultrasound technology has become so advanced in recent years that it is able to pick up more anomalies like choroid plexus cysts earlier and earlier, anomalies that statistically tend to mean nothing in most low-risk pregnancies. A meeting with a genetic counselor will help you weigh the risks and benefits of further testing in your particular situation.

Molar Pregnancy

Like an ectopic pregnancy, a molar pregnancy is also not viable. However, in a molar pregnancy, the implantation site is normal, but the embryo is not. Called a hydatidiform mole, this placental tissue develops into a mass of cysts that are often described as resembling a cluster of grapes. There are two types of molar pregnancy, complete and incomplete (or partial).

A complete molar pregnancy occurs when an egg with no genetic material inside is fertilized by one or two sperm. Most have 46 chromosomes, all from the father (paternal). The pregnancy itself contains placental mass only, and no embryonic tissue.

A partial molar pregnancy will usually contain some embryonic or fetal tissue. The majority of partial molar cases have two sets of paternal chromosomes and a single set of maternal chromosomes (69 in total).

Symptoms of molar pregnancy include:

- Too small or too large uterus for date
- Enlarged ovaries
- High hCG levels
- Vaginal bleeding
- Preeclampsia and toxemia (if diagnosis is delayed)

Ultrasound can make a definite diagnosis of molar pregnancy, which is estimated to occur in approximately one in 1,000 to 1,500 pregnancies in the United States. Older women have a higher risk for the condition, and the risk of subsequent molar pregnancy increases with each occurrence.

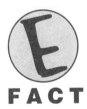

FACT

Risk of molar pregnancy is also influenced by geography. While the incidence of the condition in the United States is relatively low, about one in 120 pregnancies in Southeastern Asia is molar. Several studies have also shown a higher incidence of molar pregnancy among women in the Philippines and Mexico. The exact reasons behind this phenomenon aren't completely understood, although genetic factors, diet, and environment have all been proposed as possible influences.

Removal by dilation and curettage (D & C) is the typical treatment for molar pregnancy. D & C is a surgical procedure involving dilating the cervix and suctioning the contents of the uterus. Synthetic hormones (oxytocin) may also be administered during the procedure to induce uterine contractions.

A molar pregnancy has the potential to develop into a rare type of cancer known as choriocarcinoma. Once the D & C procedure is complete, the uterine materials are examined by a trained pathologist to ensure that they are not malignant. A chest X-ray and other radiological exams can determine if any malignancies have metastasized (spread to other parts of the body).

Follow-up blood tests may be required for 6 months to a year afterward to ensure that hCG levels have returned to normal. Levels that fail to return to normal, or start to rise, are an indication that persistent gestational trophoblastic disease (GTD) is present and further treatment is necessary. Rarely, GTD may develop into the cancerous form—metastatic choriocarcinoma. To accurately screen for these possibilities and ensure an early diagnosis, subsequent pregnancy should be avoided until the follow-up period is complete. Survival and remission rates are good if GTD is caught early and treated appropriately.

Gestational Diabetes

Gestational diabetes mellitus, or diabetes of pregnancy, is caused by a problem processing the glucose (or blood sugar) in your bloodstream. Glucose is important to the body—it provides fuel for cellular growth and metabolism. To be processed effectively, glucose requires a companion hormone known as insulin. Insulin facilitates the transfer of glucose into the cells where it is metabolized, or processed for energy. Not enough insulin, or insulin that the body isn't using effectively, and the result is a back up of glucose into the bloodstream, a situation that is potentially damaging to all of your organ systems and a developing fetus.

When you develop gestational diabetes, your pancreas is still making plenty of insulin, but your body isn't processing it efficiently. The condition, known as insulin resistance, is caused by certain placental hormones that counteract the effect of insulin (e.g., estrogen, cortisol, and human placental lactogen, or HPL). In most women, the condition doesn't reach critical levels, and their blood sugar levels stay within normal ranges. In others, excess blood glucose accumulates to potentially dangerous levels and treatment is required.

The Odds

Gestational diabetes mellitus (GDM) occurs in up to 7 percent of all pregnancies in the United States. Factors that may make you more likely to develop GDM include obesity, a family history of diabetes, a diagnosis of GDM or large birth weight babies in previous pregnancies, and being over age 25.

Diagnosis and Treatment

Diagnosis of GDM is made with the glucose tolerance test (GTT). See Chapter 5 for details on how the GTT is performed.

Because blood sugar levels are influenced by dietary intake, your provider will probably try to treat your GDM with lifestyle and nutritional changes at the onset. A visit with a certified diabetes educator (CDE) and a registered dietitian (RD) can be invaluable in learning more about healthy menu planning, exercise, and the basics of blood sugar control.

You will have to self-test your blood glucose levels on a regular basis with a home meter. The home meter uses a lancet to prick your finger, arm, or another test site for a blood sample. The blood droplet is placed on a test reagent strip that goes into the meter, and the meter provides a blood glucose reading. Testing is generally recommended first thing in the morning (a fasting test), and after meals (postprandial)—usually at 1 hour and again at 2 hours after eating. Your doctor may recommend testing at additional times, such as after exercise, if he feels it is warranted. Refer to the table to see what blood glucose levels the American Diabetes Association recommends for women with gestational diabetes.

If you don't experience significant improvement with dietary changes and your glucose levels still exceed normal ranges, you may have to take insulin injections to keep your blood sugar under control. Injections are typically taken before meals to counteract their impact on glucose levels. Insulin does not cross the placenta and is not harmful to fetal development.

Blood Glucose Levels in Women with Gestational Diabetes	
Test	Range
Fasting whole blood glucose	<95 mg/dl (5.3 mmol/l)*
Fasting plasma glucose	<105 mg/dl (5.8 mmol/l)
1 hour postprandial whole blood glucose	<140 mg/dl (7.8 mmol/l)
1 hour postprandial plasma glucose	<155 mg/dl (8.6 mmol/l)
2 hour postprandial whole blood glucose	<120 mg/dl (6.7 mmol/l)
2 hour postprandial plasma glucose	<130 mg/dl (7.2 mmol/l)

*Note: mg/dl is the U.S. unit of measure for blood glucose readings, and mmol/l is the international measurement. Most home meters use plasma readings, the same as at your doctor's office, but some are still calibrated to whole blood, so both measurements are provided.

Possible Long-Term Health Effects

Without proper treatment, uncontrolled blood glucose levels can result in fetal death or a condition known as fetal macrosomia (a baby that is too large). Blood glucose crosses the placenta in high levels and the fetus responds by producing more insulin to process the load. The extra glucose is ultimately stored as fat, and the baby potentially grows too large for vaginal birth.

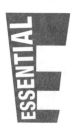

Women who develop gestational diabetes have an increased risk of a diagnosis of type 2 diabetes later in life, and should receive regular screening for the disease. Their children are also at risk for both type 2 diabetes and obesity. Fortunately, clinical studies have also shown that lifestyle changes involving regular exercise and a healthy diet can be extremely effective in preventing the onset of type 2 diabetes.

Newborns of GDM moms may also suffer from hypoglycemia (or low blood sugar) at birth as they are suddenly "disconnected" from the maternal surge of glucose and their high insulin production causes their blood glucose levels to plummet. They may also have an imbalance of blood calcium and blood magnesium levels at birth. Because of these risks, a neonatologist may be on the scene during labor and delivery to treat any potential complications.

Hyperemesis Gravidarum

Hyperemesis gravidarum is excessive nausea and vomiting of pregnancy (i.e., morning sickness) that goes beyond the normal gastrointestinal disturbance experienced by many women. Its exact cause is unknown. The condition is diagnosed when nausea and vomiting trigger one or more of the following symptoms:

- Weight loss of 10 pounds or more
- Ketosis
- Dehydration
- Electrolyte imbalance

Other conditions that can cause similar symptoms—including hyperthyroidism, pancreatitis, gall bladder or liver disease, gastritis, appendicitis, and ectopic pregnancy—should be ruled out before diagnosing *hyperemesis gravidarum*. Treatment typically involves intravenous therapy to rehydrate and encourage weight gain (parenteral nutrition). Hospitalization may be required, and medications may also be prescribed.

Fortunately, *hyperemesis gravidarum* is relatively uncommon, occurring in up to 10 of every 1,000 pregnancies. For more on nausea and vomiting in pregnancy, see Chapter 2.

Incompetent Cervix

An incompetent cervix is a cervix that starts to open (efface and/or dilate) prematurely. It may be caused by a multiple pregnancy (twins or more), genetic factors, prior surgeries, or a history of abortion. If your mother took the drug DES (diethylstilbestrol) when she was pregnant with you, you may also be at risk for an incompetent cervix.

As pregnancy progresses and your unborn child grows and places more pressure on the cervix, an incompetent cervix may result in miscarriage without treatment. Women who have had problems with incompetent cervix in previous pregnancies, or are considered at risk due to multiples, may be regularly monitored using transvaginal ultrasound to detect any cervical changes. If you ever experience vaginal bleeding or blood-tinged discharge, let your provider know immediately.

Surgery to suture (stitch) the cervix closed, called a cerclage, may be recommended to prevent premature cervical opening. There are several different methods of cerclage, including the Shirodkar, the McDonald, and abdominal cerclage. The most common type, the McDonald, is a temporary suture that is removed when labor begins. Another treatment option may be an appliance called a pessary, which is inserted into your vagina to support your cervix and uterus. Finally, bed rest may be prescribed to keep weight off your uterus, and abstinence from sexual intercourse will probably be recommended.

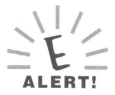

ALERT!

DES daughters, or women who were exposed to the drug DES (diethylstilbestrol) while in their mother's womb, are at risk for an array of health problems. If your mother was treated with DES (which she may be familiar with as synthetic estrogen) between 1940 and 1971, particularly in the first 5 months of pregnancy, the drug may have affected the development of your reproductive organs. DES daughters are at a higher risk for miscarriage, preterm birth, ectopic pregnancy, and a rare form of cancer called clear cell adenocarcinoma.

Intrauterine Growth Restriction (IUGR)

Intrauterine growth restriction (IUGR) occurs when fetal weight and size gain are estimated to be below the tenth percentile for gestational age. Some IUGR babies may be preterm, but others go to full term. IUGR occurs in up to 10 percent of pregnancies.

Possible causes of IUGR include the following.

- **Multiple gestations.** IUGR occurs in at least one fetus in up to 20 percent of twins or higher order multiples pregnancies.
- **Infection.** Infectious agents such as toxoplasmosis and cytomegalovirus.
- **Placental problems.** Placenta previa, accreta, or abruption, along with other placental abnormalities.
- **Umbilical cord compression.** Knots or twisting may decrease fetal blood supply.
- **Maternal hypertension.** High blood pressure in pregnancy, including preeclampsia.
- **Maternal tobacco, alcohol, and drug use.** Smoking moms-to-be are almost twice as likely as non-smokers to have a low-birthweight baby.
- **Poor maternal nutrition.** Malnutrition and inadequate protein intake can restrict fetal growth and may lead to adult health problems such as hypertension and insulin resistance later in life.
- **Genetic anomalies.** Arrested physical and mental growth is one of the features of many chromosomal disorders, including Down Syndrome and Edwards Syndrome (Trisomy 21 and Trisomy 18).
- **Birth defect.** Birth defects such as a congenital heart or kidney malformation may restrict blood flow and affect fetal growth.
- **Altitude.** The reduced oxygen supply at high elevations decreases blood flow to the uterus and placenta, and is thought to be a factor in IUGR and low birth weight.
- **Certain chronic illnesses.** Maternal heart disease, sickle cell disease, diabetes, and systemic lupus erythematosis (SLE, or lupus), among others.

A fundal height (uterus height) that is measuring too small for the due date is the first tip-off to IUGR. An ultrasound can give your provider an idea of actual fetal size, and if IUGR is diagnosed you will probably be undergoing regular ultrasounds, non-stress tests, and biophysical profiles through the remainder of pregnancy to follow your baby's progress (see Chapter 5 for more information on these procedures).

IUGR pregnancies are at risk for intrapartum asphyxia (blocked oxygen flow to fetus), oligohydramnios (low amniotic fluid volume), and possible preterm birth and its related complications. At birth, IUGR babies are at risk for a number of medical problems, including high blood pressure, hypoglycemia (low blood sugar), anemia, polycythemia (an excess of red blood cells), neurological problems, and jaundice. Later in life they may experience some developmental problems. Low birth weight (LBW), including both IUGR and preterm LBW, is the leading cause of infant mortality in the United States.

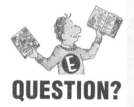

QUESTION?

What's the difference between IUGR and a preterm baby?
Preterm babies are typically also low birth weight (LBW), but they are still considered the appropriate size for their actual gestational age (time spent in the womb). Newborns diagnosed with intra-uterine growth restriction, on the other hand, may be born at full term and *still* be small for gestational age (SGA). So in an acronym nutshell, non-IUGR preterm babies are LBW but not SGA, while IUGR babies (which can be preterm or full-term) are both LBW and SGA.

IUGR that begins early in pregnancy and affects the fetal body uniformly is said to be symmetric. Symmetric IUGR may be caused by genetic abnormality, fetal infection, or exposure to teratogen. Growth restriction that occurs later in pregnancy and is thought to be caused by insufficient fetal nutrition is termed asymmetric IUGR. It is also called head sparing IUGR because the fetus has focused its limited resources on vital brain development, making the head in these babies much larger than the body. Asymmetric IUGR infants typically have a better prognosis, or long-term outlook.

Placenta Problems

The placenta provides nourishment, blood, and oxygen to your baby, and is literally what connects the two of you. Problems can occur with either the structure or the placement of the placenta, which may pose a risk to you and your unborn child.

Uteroplacental Insufficiency (UPI)

Uteroplacental insufficiency occurs when the blood flow, and consequently oxygen supply, from mother to fetus is impaired or inadequate in some way. This is usually the result of an acute or chronic maternal illness (e.g., hypertension, diabetes, preeclampsia, kidney disease), although it can arise from chromosomal abnormalities in the fetus. It may also occur in cases of multiple gestation (i.e., twins, triplets, or more).

Clinical signs that UPI may be present include:

- **Oligohydramnios.** Low levels of amniotic fluid, apparent on ultrasound.
- **A nonreactive non-stress test (NST).** If the fetus is hypoxic (getting insufficient oxygen), its heart rate will not accelerate with, or react to, fetal movement.
- **Late decelerations in a stress test (or contraction stress test).** A slowdown in fetal heart rate that peaks toward the end of a contraction also indicates hypoxia.
- **Intrauterine growth restriction (IUGR; see above).** A fetus that is small for gestational age on ultrasound.

If you are diagnosed with UPI, steps will be taken to correct or treat the underlying cause if possible. Fetal distress may be cause for immediate caesarean delivery.

Placenta Previa

A placenta that implants and grows near or covering the cervical opening, or os, occurs in up to 20 percent of pregnancies in the second trimester. This condition, called placenta previa, often resolves itself by moving upward and away from the os about 90 percent of the time. However, if placenta previa persists late in pregnancy, potentially life-threatening hemorrhage can occur when the cervix starts to efface (thin) if the placenta separates prematurely.

Placenta previa may be total (i.e., completely covering the os), partial (i.e., partially covering the os), or marginal (i.e., on the margin, or edge, of the os). The condition is diagnosed by ultrasound. Vaginal bleeding is a possible symptom, but some women have no symptoms whatsoever.

If bleeding does occur, bed rest may be prescribed. Blood transfusion may also be necessary. Women who have a complete placenta previa will require a caesarean delivery. Those with a partial or marginal placenta previa can potentially deliver vaginally, but both the patient and the provider should be prepared for an emergency C-section if required.

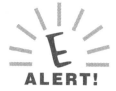

ALERT!

A low-lying placenta is a placenta that is near to the os, but not close enough to be considered marginal. Like placenta previa, this type of placental implantation has a higher risk of separation during late pregnancy.

Placental Abruption

Vaginal bleeding, abdominal cramping, and symptoms of shock (i.e., irregular heartbeat, low blood pressure, pale complexion) can signal that the placenta has begun to prematurely separate from the wall of the uterus, a condition called placental abruption (or *abruptio placenta*). Risk factors for placental abruption include maternal high blood pressure, cocaine use, or physical trauma to the abdomen.

Abruption may occur anytime after week 20, and if you have had a previous occurrence in an earlier pregnancy, your risk of experiencing it again is increased. Placental abruption may cause major life-threatening hemorrhage, fetal distress or possibly death, and preterm labor. However, a swift diagnosis and initiation of treatment, including blood transfusion, IV fluids, and oxygen, can do much to improve outcomes. Immediate delivery, possibly by C-section, will be indicated in the majority of cases, but depends on the stability of both mother and fetus and the length of gestation.

Placenta Accreta

Placenta accreta occurs when the placenta implants or attaches to the myometrium, or uterine muscle, instead of the endometrium. Placenta accreta can be further categorized into two subtypes based on the extent of myometrium invasion—placenta increta and placenta percreta.

In pregnancy complicated by placenta accreta, the placenta does not easily separate from the uterine wall during the third stage of delivery, and hemorrhage occurs. A postpartum blood transfusion, arterial embolization, or an emergency hysterectomy (surgical removal of the uterus) may be required to stop the bleeding and stabilize the patient. If you are diagnosed with this condition prior to delivery, it's important to discuss the possibility of a hysterectomy. In some clinical situations, a hysterectomy may be unavoidable, but if an option is available, your doctor needs to know of any desire for more children so he can preserve your fertility if at all possible.

According to the ACOG, the incidence of placenta accreta has risen dramatically in the past 50 years and currently happens at a rate of one of every 2,500 deliveries. This increase can probably be traced to the climb in caesarean section rates; placenta accreta is more likely to occur in women with a history of caesarean delivery (and climbs with each subsequent C-section). In addition, women who were diagnosed with placenta previa in previous pregnancies have a substantially increased risk of placenta accreta.

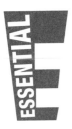

If you are considered at risk for the condition, magnetic resonance imaging (MRI) and ultrasound may be used to confirm a diagnosis. A high alpha-fetoprotein (AFP) level may also be a sign of placenta accreta. See Chapter 5 for more details on these diagnostic tests.

Preeclampsia/Toxemia/Eclampsia

Pregnancy induced hypertension (PIH), or otherwise uncomplicated high blood pressure of pregnancy occurring after 20 weeks gestation, appears in up to 10 percent of pregnancies. A condition called preeclampsia (or toxemia) happens in 5 to 7 percent of pregnancies and is characterized by the following symptoms:

- High blood pressure (140/90 or higher)
- Excessive swelling of hands and/or feet

- Sudden weight gain
- Protein in the urine
- Blurry vision
- Abdominal pain
- Headache

Preeclampsia may be controlled by bed rest, medication, and careful monitoring of the fetus. Hospitalization may be required. If the pregnancy has reached 37 weeks, delivery may be induced or performed via C-section to avoid further risk.

When preeclampsia does not improve with treatment, or goes undiagnosed, it may develop into eclampsia, a rare but potentially life-threatening condition where convulsions occur.

Premature Labor

Delivery of your baby after week 24 and before week 37 of pregnancy is considered preterm or premature. In cases of very early preterm labor where fetal lung maturity hasn't been established, your provider will probably try to delay the delivery for as long as possible. Preemies can suffer from a wide range of physical, neurological, and developmental difficulties, so any extra time spent in the womb is beneficial.

Are You At Risk?

A number of environmental and physical factors can increase your chance of preterm delivery. These include, but are not limited to:

- Previous premature labor
- Pregnant with multiples (twins or more)
- Previous uterine surgery
- Hypertension (high blood pressure)
- Cigarette smoking
- Diagnosed incompetent cervix
- Drug or alcohol abuse
- Vaginal or systemic infection

- Exposure to drug diethylstilbestrol (DES)
- Preterm, premature rupture of membranes (PPROM)

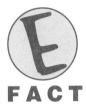

FACT

A clinical study of women at high risk for premature birth found that injections of a form of the hormone progesterone administered in the second and third trimesters cut the risk of preterm labor by up to 42 percent. Data from the study, which was sponsored by the National Institute of Child Health and Human Development (NICHD), was presented at the 23rd Annual Meeting of the Society for Maternal Fetal Medicine in February 2003. The drug—which is called 17-alpha-hydroxyprogesterone caproate—is approved by the FDA as a progestin.

Warning Signs

If you experience any of the following warning signs of preterm labor, call your health care provider immediately. If you are out of town or unable to get in touch with her for any reason, go directly to the nearest hospital emergency room. With prompt action, it may be possible to delay your labor until your unborn child has adequate time to develop.

Symptoms include:

- Painful contractions at regular intervals
- Abdominal cramps
- Lower backache
- Bloody vaginal discharge
- Stomach pain
- Any type of fluid leak from the vagina, large or small

Treatment

Preterm labor may be halted by bed rest, tocolytic medications (drugs that stop contractions), and intravenous hydration. Depending on your medical history and how far along your pregnancy is, you may be hospitalized. Home bed rest may also be prescribed, and you may be required to hook up to a fetal monitor on a regular basis. If preterm labor occurs between 24 and 34 weeks, corticosteroids may be administered to hasten fetal lung surfactant development, as well.

If your cervix dilates to 4 or 5 centimeters, or if your fetus is showing signs of distress, preterm delivery may be unavoidable.

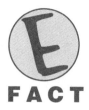

FACT

A level-three neonatal intensive care unit (NICU) is the best place for your newborn to receive treatment if he or she is delivered preterm. These units are highly experienced in the care of high-risk newborns and preemies and have state-of-the-art technology and training. A 1996 study published in the *Journal of the American Medical Association* found that level-three NICUs were associated with a 38 percent reduction in high-risk infant mortality compared to hospitals without an NICU. For more information on spending time in the NICU, see Chapter 7.

Preterm Premature Rupture of Membranes (PPROM)

Premature rupture of the amniotic membrane is not necessarily a problem if it occurs late in pregnancy. However, when it happens before week 37 of gestation, certain steps should be taken to ensure your fetus has enough time for development in the womb.

PPROM may occur in women at risk for preterm labor. Other possible causes of PPROM include cervical incompetence and vaginal infection. If PPROM occurs prior to 37 weeks, bed rest and frequent fetal heart monitoring may be undertaken in an effort to prolong pregnancy until the fetal lungs mature. Antibiotics are administered to ward off infection in both fetus and mother, and steroids may be prescribed to speed lung surfactant production in the fetus.

Bed Rest

If you're experiencing a medical condition that puts you at risk for pre-term labor, your provider may send you to your room—for strict bed rest.

Why Bed Rest May Be Necessary

Bed rest takes the forces of gravity off your cervix, gives your circulatory system and blood pressure a break, and has the added benefit of promoting rest and stress reduction.

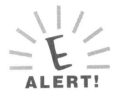
ALERT!

Amniotic fluid that is greenish or brown in color may contain meconium, your baby's first bowel movement. The presence of meconium can indicate fetal distress, as the tarry substance may be aspirated (inhaled) in the womb. If you are leaking amniotic fluid and there are signs of meconium, the situation should be evaluated by your provider immediately.

Staying Sane

At first, that bed may seem like a welcome oasis, particularly if you've been getting little sleep as of late. A prescription to snooze! What more could you ask for?

That feeling will likely be short-lived, however. There's only so much you can do horizontally (or even slightly tilted). Yet there are ways to make the time pass a little faster. Some ideas to keep busy beyond the usual TV and rental movie fare:

- **Baby shopping by mail or modem.** Get on your laptop or leaf through some of those catalogs your mailbox has been inundated with. Shopping has never been so easy on your feet.
- **Get crafty.** Creating something special for baby—embroidered, crocheted, or knitted—is a good way to pass the hours. Even if you are a rookie, a beginner's kit can get you started. You may not have the time again for years, so go for it.
- **Feed your mind.** Read, read, read. Not just baby books (although feel free to keep this one handy), but classics, new fiction, and anything else you can get your hands on.
- **Catch up.** All those pictures you've been meaning to put into photo albums, the scrapbooks that are half finished, letters on your list to

write, and other assorted undertakings are perfect bed rest projects that have the added bonus of imparting a sense of achievement.

- **Be game.** Dust off some of those old board and strategy games you haven't played in years, and recruit your partner or kids to play, too. A rousing game of Risk can be a lot more entertaining than another evening spent channel surfing.

Miscarriage

Up to 20 percent of all detected pregnancies miscarry before 20 weeks of gestation. Also referred to as spontaneous abortion or missed abortion, about half the time miscarriages are caused by chromosomal abnormalities, or what's known as a blighted ovum—a fertilized egg that implants but does not develop into an embryo.

Other factors to be considered in a miscarriage are:

- Hormonal deficiencies
- Abnormalities of the cervix or uterus
- Incompatible blood types or the Rh factor
- Viruses and infections
- Immune disorders

Warning Signs

Some of the warning signs of miscarriage can also happen in perfectly normal and healthy pregnancies. Light blood spotting, for example, is a common occurrence in pregnancy when implantation takes place and may occur throughout the first trimester.

Better safe than sorry is always the rule in pregnancy, however. Do take any symptoms seriously and contact your provider as soon as they occur, but keep in mind that the appearance of blood spots or minor cramping doesn't guarantee miscarriage.

Signs and symptoms of miscarriage may include:

- Bright red vaginal bleeding
- Abdominal cramping

- Low back pain
- High fever
- Extreme nausea and vomiting that's sudden and unusual
- Amniotic fluid leakage
- Severe headache

Some women panic when they experience a sudden improvement in previously troublesome pregnancy symptoms. Remember that this is a common phenomenon toward the end of the first trimester as hormone levels start to balance out. If you're still concerned, or something just doesn't feel quite right, call your provider to schedule a quick appointment for a listen to the fetal heartbeat. Most will be happy to comply to ease your mind.

Coping with Loss

It doesn't take long to fall hopelessly in love with your unborn child, to dream about your future together, and to start making a special place within your family for him or her. "Love at first thought" is perhaps the most accurate way to describe how many moms and dads feel about it.

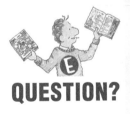

QUESTION?

We lost a baby, our first, to miscarriage last year. Is there anything we can do to prevent it this time around?
Many miscarriages occur due to factors completely beyond anyone's control—a defective egg or sperm, implantation outside of the endometrium. Other triggers, such as teratogen exposure, may be avoided with special precautions in pregnancy. Definitely speak with your health care provider about your concerns and any special instructions given your medical history (e.g., activity restrictions).

That is what makes pregnancy loss so difficult at any point in the process. You may hear insensitive comments like, "Well, at least you were only a few weeks along," that are meant to be sympathetic but only serve to minimize the very real grief you are experiencing. Give yourself adequate time to mourn, and to deal with the feelings of anger, guilt, frustration, and depression. Talk to your doctor about a referral to a pregnancy loss support group or a one-on-one counselor or therapist. You may also want to visit the Hygeia Foundation for Perinatal Loss, Inc., for online support and information at ✑ *www.hygeia.org*.

It's extremely important to take care of yourself during this difficult time. If you hadn't yet told anyone about the pregnancy at the point miscarriage occurred, it may be tougher to find enough time to reflect and grieve. Allow yourself to take a few sick or personal days off from work to spend healing time with your significant other and family. Don't rush things.

Trying Again

When to try again is a delicate issue. You need to be ready both emotionally and physically. Make sure you have had time to grieve your loss, and consult with your provider about the causes behind your first miscarriage. Your provider might recommend that you wait for a period to allow your body time to recover. If you do want to try again immediately, make sure you express your wishes so you both can prepare properly for the next time around.

If you've experienced repeated miscarriage, considered clinically to be three consecutive pregnancy losses before 20 weeks, further investigation will be in order before attempting another pregnancy. The cause can sometimes be determined by a pathological examination of the miscarried fetus or embryo. A meeting with a genetic counselor, and a full pre-conception diagnostic workup to examine your fallopian tubes, uterus, and other possible sites of a problem, may also be recommended. Ⓔ

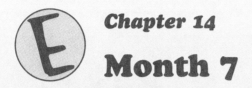

Chapter 14

Month 7

I t's the home stretch, the final act, the big countdown—the third trimester. You've made a lot of decisions so far, and there are even more to be made this month. Full speed ahead with labor and delivery preparations this month as you schedule childbirth classes and start to assemble a birth plan.

Baby This Month

Weighing in at 4 pounds and about 16 inches long, your baby is growing amazingly fast now. Her red, wrinkled skin is losing its fine lanugo covering as more insulating fat accumulates. And her eyelids, closed for so long, can now open and afford her a dim view of the place she will call home for just a few more months.

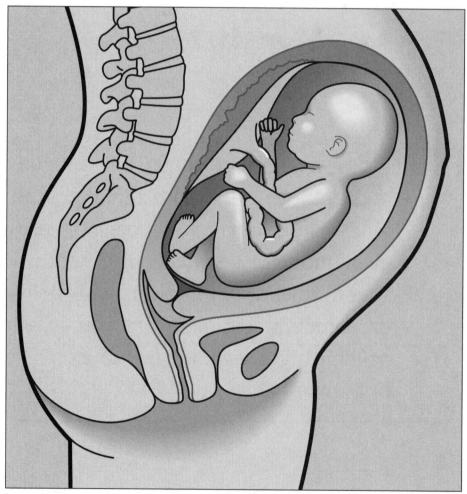

▲ You and your baby as you kick off the third trimester.

Dramatic developments in the brain and central nervous system are also occurring, as baby's nerve cells are sheathed with a substance called myelin that speeds nerve impulses. A 7-month-old fetus feels pain, can cry, and responds to stimulation from light or sound outside the womb.

Her gymnastics may subside as her space gets smaller, but you're feeling her more intensely now and her movements may even be visible to both you and your partner. Periodically, tiny elbows and feet will turn your belly into an interactive relief map. Gently pushing back can provide endless entertainment for all three of you. You've heard about it, now play the game at home—it's "Name That Body Part."

Even though your fetus is still producing lung surfactant and developing alveoli (air sacs), her lungs still aren't developed enough to breathe in the outside world. If complications required an early delivery now, steroids might be administered intravenously to boost surfactant production. Chemical surfactants can also be used after birth to help with respiratory distress.

Your Body This Month

You're likely feeling perpetually stuffed and slightly out of breath as your uterus relocates all your internal organs. The relief and energy felt in the second trimester may start to fade now. Just remember, you're almost there!

Your Body Changes

The top of the fundus is halfway between your belly button and your breastbone, displacing your stomach, intestines, and diaphragm. Your expanding abdomen has formed a shelf, handy for resting your arms on and balancing a cold beverage at the movies. On the downside, you'll be catching a lot of crumbs, and your napkin just doesn't seem to stay on your lap anymore.

Not only are your breasts heavier, but also they are more glandular and getting ready to feed your baby. In this last trimester, your nipples may begin to leak colostrum, which is the yellowish, nutrient-rich fluid that precedes real breast milk. You may find the leaking more apparent when you're sexually aroused. To reduce backaches and breast tenderness, make sure you wear a well-fitting bra (even to bed if it helps). If you are planning on breastfeeding, you may want to consider buying some supportive nursing bras now that can take you through the rest of pregnancy and right into the postpartum period.

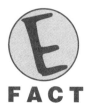

FACT

If you're picking up some nursing bras, be sure to test-drive the clasps for easy nursing access. Try to unfasten and slip the nursing flaps down with one hand. This may seem unimportant now, but when you're in the middle of a crowded shopping mall juggling packages and trying to discreetly put baby to breast single-handedly, you'll be thankful you had the foresight.

What You Feel Like

Your body is warming up for labor, and you may start to experience Braxton-Hicks contractions. These painless and irregular contractions feel as if your uterus is making a fist and then gradually relaxing it. If your little one is fairly active, you may think that she is stretching herself sideways at first. A quick check of your belly may reveal a visible tightening.

Braxton-Hicks can begin as early as week 20 and continue right up until your due date, although they're more commonly felt in the final month of pregnancy. Some first-time moms-to-be are afraid they won't be able to tell the difference between Braxton-Hicks and actual labor contractions. As any woman who has been through labor will attest, when the real thing comes you'll know it. Rule of thumb: If it hurts, it's labor.

Starting at week 20, the uterus has a basic rhythm. The smooth muscle of the uterus is similar to your intestinal tract in that both involuntarily contract in a wavelike pattern designed to facilitate movement of what's inside (be it breakfast or your baby). These early rhythmic and generally painless contractions are called Braxton-Hicks when they do not cause any changes to the cervix and occur at irregular intervals. They may even be uncomfortable at times, but will usually subside if you change positions, another way to distinguish Braxton-Hicks from the real thing. The actual definition of labor, even when it is premature, is the onset of regular, painful, uterine contractions that lead to a change in the cervix.

If your contractions suddenly seem to be coming at regular intervals and they start to cause you pain or discomfort, they may be the real thing. Lie down on your left side for about a half-hour with a clock or watch on hand, and time the contractions from the beginning of one to the beginning of the next. If the interludes are more or less regular, call your health care provider. And if contractions of any type are accompanied by blood or amniotic fluid leakage, contact your practitioner immediately.

The list is growing. Other symptoms that may continue this month include:

- Fatigue
- Frequent urination
- Tender and/or swollen breasts
- Bleeding gums
- Excess mucus and saliva
- Increase in normal vaginal discharge
- Mild shortness of breath
- Lightheadedness or dizziness
- Headaches
- Forgetfulness
- Gas, heartburn, and/or constipation
- Skin and hair changes
- Round ligament pain or soreness
- Lower back aches
- Mild swelling of legs, feet, and hands
- Leg cramps

At the Doctor

Starting with this initial third-trimester visit, your visits to the doctor may start to step up to twice monthly. Your provider will probably want to know if you've been experiencing any Braxton-Hicks contractions, and he will cover the warning signs of preterm labor and what you should do if you experience them (read more on preterm labor in Chapter 13). If you're unsure about what type of childbirth class you'd like to take, you might want to bring your questions to your provider for her take. Just remember, the decision is ultimately up to you and your partner.

Women who are Rh negative will need treatment with Rh immune globulin (RhoGAM) this month. An injection is typically given at about 28 weeks to protect the fetus from developing hemolytic disease—a condition in which the mother's antibodies attack the fetal red blood cells.

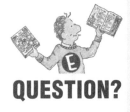

QUESTION?

Why is everyone always touching me, and how can I get them to stop?
People are fascinated with the life force of pregnancy, and you're radiating it big time. While your family is granted fairly open access to your belly, coworkers and acquaintances are another story. To fend off the feelers who ask permission first, simply tell them you're somewhat sensitive about your stomach right now. You may have a tougher time stopping those swoopers who strike without warning, but if you can anticipate their moves you might be able to block with a step back or a turn away. Hopefully, they'll get the hint.

On Your Mind

This month will bring new questions and uncertainties as you ponder your ideal birth experience. Are you looking forward to a completely chemical-free birth, or are you already exploring your pain-killing options? Is your provider open to your needs and willing to make reasonable accommodations to meet them? Do you want only your partner in attendance or would you like additional support? Whatever your perfect labor and delivery is, make sure the direction of your birth plan is driven by the needs of you and your partner and not by the expectations of others.

Keep in mind that you don't want to create such incredibly high expectations of yourself and of the experience that you're bound to be let down. Try to build in room for flexibility in your conception of the ultimate birth. Your little one may not be following the same game plan as you, and last-minute strategy changes are often required. Luckily, if you work on your birth plan now you can make allowances for complications within it and save yourself unnecessary angst later. Turn ahead to Chapter 15 for tips on putting together your birth plan.

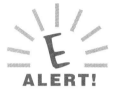

ALERT!

Don't miss the boat on insurance. Many childbirth classes, sibling classes, and breastfeeding classes are completely covered by your health insurance provider. If cost is holding you back, check out your coverage. Even if you aren't covered, courses are usually relatively inexpensive and many facilities offer sliding-fee scales for those who qualify.

Childbirth Classes

Most childbirth seminars available through hospitals and birthing centers are called prepared childbirth classes. Taking place in a classroom setting, and using lectures, audiovisuals, and floor exercises to get you ready for labor and delivery, prepared childbirth classes may focus on one, two, or more birth philosophies. They may vary in length from several months of Saturdays to a one-day seminar. While hospital policy will dictate a lot of what's covered, here's a general idea of what you will experience:

- **Commiseration.** You'll interact with other pregnant couples and demonstrate that misery (and joy) truly does love company.
- **Reality.** Through lecture and (in many cases) actual video footage, you'll get the full scoop on what really goes on in labor and delivery.
- **Guided tour.** If your class is at the birthing center or hospital, you will probably get a tour of the facilities and some basic instructions on when and where to show up when labor hits. The best part? The nursery window stop, of course.
- **Teamwork.** Your husband, partner, or labor coach will learn more about his or her role in this process, and you may even be given homework to try out techniques at home.
- **After-birth instruction.** Many classes offer valuable information on breastfeeding basics and baby care. Don't be surprised if the instructor brings in a bag full of baby dolls for practice.

- **Seasoned support.** Most prepared childbirth classes will be conducted by a trained childbirth educator.
- **Paperwork.** More literature, brochures, pamphlets, handouts, forms, photocopies, and leaflets will come your way. Bring a bag.

Perhaps the most important facet of childbirth class, and certainly the one that most first-time moms pay the closest attention to, is the information it provides on managing labor and delivery discomforts. In addition to an overview of anesthesia and pain medication options, childbirth educators may draw on one or more childbirth philosophies to teach coping methods. Some of the most popular and widely taught techniques are outlined below.

Lamaze Method

Lamaze, or psychoprophylaxis, is probably the most well-known childbirth method in use in the United States today. Named after Dr. Fernand Lamaze, classes are taught by certified Lamaze instructors and attended by more than two million parents-to-be annually.

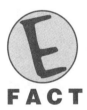

FACT

Dr. Fernand Lamaze came up with the kernel of his theories on painless prepared childbirth after a trip to Russia in the early 1950s, which familiarized him with the works of Ivan Pavlov. If the name sounds familiar, you probably remember Pavlov from Psych 101—he's the Nobel-winning behavioral scientist behind the famed drooling dogs, which were conditioned to equate the sound of a bell with their dinner.

If you've never been in a Lamaze class, you probably equate the name with heavy, hyperventilated breathing. True Lamaze classes, however, are much more than panting practice. While rhythmic breathing exercises are stressed for each stage of labor in Lamaze, helpful laboring and birth positions, relaxation techniques, and pain management are also covered. In addition to massage, water therapy, and hot and cold compresses, you're taught how to focus on a picture or object to diminish your discomfort.

Lamaze is founded on the principle that instinct and what Lamaze International calls "inner wisdom" guide women through the birth process. Lamaze also stresses the empowerment of the mother-to-be and her right to the birth experience and environment she wants.

Bradley Method

Denver obstetrician Robert Bradley, the author of *Husband Coached Childbirth,* developed this popular approach to labor and delivery. As you may have guessed, he was a big advocate of fathers helping their partners through the birth process, and in fact many consider his work instrumental in opening up the labor room door to dads.

Bradley classes teach couples how to relax and breathe deeply, but the emphasis is on doing what comes naturally—father as coach, proper nutrition during pregnancy, and most important, knowing all the options beforehand. They also emphasize the *natural* in natural childbirth, suggesting that pain medication be used as a last resort rather than a front-line tool.

Hypnobirthing and Dr. Grantly Dick-Read

British doctor and natural childbirth pioneer Grantly Dick-Read, who authored the classic *Childbirth Without Fear*, is the inspiration behind hypnobirthing education. Dick-Read believed that a woman's labor pains were magnified by her fear and anxieties. Hypnobirthing, based on Dick-Read's teachings, emphasizes slow abdominal breathing and other relaxation techniques that teach you how to focus on the feelings and signals your body sends during labor.

LeBoyer Method

Dr. Frederick LeBoyer, author of *Birth Without Violence*, developed this method of childbirth that attempts to soften the trauma of the transition from the warm, dark womb to the big bright world. It advocates dim lights in the delivery room, a warm bath for the new baby, calm voices, and soothing room temperatures.

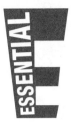

If your last pregnancy ended in a caesarean section and you're going to try to deliver vaginally this time around, inquire about a VBAC, or vaginal birth after caesarean, class. VBAC courses provide couples with information on the benefits, risks, and statistics surrounding vaginal births following a C-section. They are usually recommended as a supplement to, and not a replacement for, a prepared childbirth class.

The Right Teacher and the Right Class

Completely confused now? Don't know your Bradley from your LeBoyer? A good first step is to call your hospital or birthing center and ask for printed schedules and descriptions of upcoming classes—many of your questions will probably be answered right there. Once you get a basic feel for what is offered, you can call with follow-up questions about instructor credentials and training, methods taught, class size, curriculum, and costs. You might also ask if there are couples who have taken the course that you can contact as references.

If you find that the classes or curriculum offered at your local hospital just aren't what you're looking for, you may opt for private instruction. The International Childbirth Education Association (ICEA) can provide you with names of certified instructors in your area. You can contact the Minneapolis-based ICEA at ✆ 952-854-8660 or online at ✎ *www.icea.org.*

Touring the Hospital/Birthing Center

Even if you don't choose a childbirth class sponsored by the facility at which you'll be giving birth, you should try to arrange a tour. Getting your bearings ahead of time will save you valuable time and frustration when the big day arrives. If you're in the middle of the mother-of-all contractions, the last thing you want to do is try to figure out where validated parking is. You'll also have less anxiety and disappointment if you know what to expect of the labor and birthing rooms. What you imagine (a flower-filled, sunny room filled with soft music and framed watercolors) may be a far cry from reality.

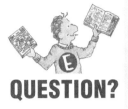

QUESTION?

The childbirth educator mentioned having a pediatrician for our baby. Isn't it too early for that?
On the contrary, now is the perfect time to interview prospective candidates. Your pediatrician will look in on and care for your newborn in the hospital, so getting one lined up now is important. Some things to inquire about beyond the basic office hours and insurance questions—do ill children have a separate waiting room than those who are there for well-child visits; will the doctor support your feeding choice; are lactation consultants available; and how are calls into the office triaged and returned?

Classes for Siblings

New sibling classes can be a huge boon for parents who are on their second pregnancy. Typically divided by age group so information can be communicated at an appropriate level, these classes put an emphasis on the emotional side of having a new family member—how things at home are changing, how the family will adjust after baby is born, and what they're feeling about these developments.

There's also plenty of practical information provided, including a preview tour of mom's accommodations and some basic big brother/ sister baby-handling guidelines. Even the youngest kids are usually given the opportunity to "practice" baby care with a doll.

If your child is having difficulty adjusting to the idea of a new baby in the house, a sibling class can make him feel more involved in, and consequently more accepting of, your family's growth. As you might imagine, the ability of the instructor to relate to your child can make or break this type of class, so getting a few referrals may be time well spent. If you have the opportunity, you might inquire about the possibility of spending 15 minutes in the back of an upcoming class to test the waters before sending your child to participate.

See Appendix A for more information resources on childbirth education.

Just for Dads

Depending on today's viewpoint, the light, or the fire, at the end of the tunnel is becoming brighter. In 3 months, you will be witnessing your child's first breath in this world. Although your partner will be doing the grunt work, you'll need to start studying your role in this final drama as (A) a shoulder to lean on; (B) a forgiving target to vent at; and (C) head cheerleader.

About Childbirth Classes

If you are the type that thrives on clear instructions and routine, you may find the idea of childbirth class a port in the pregnancy storm. "Woo hoo!" you think, "At last someone is going to tell me what to do." Well, not quite. Yes, you will be taught techniques you can use to help your partner through labor and delivery, and you'll learn in graphic detail just how that baby is going to get from point A to point B. But you aren't getting any step-by-step instructions or checklists that are money-back guaranteed to get you from the first contraction to, "It's a boy/girl!" Labor and delivery is not a math problem or a computer program. Your best preparation is to be ready for the unexpected.

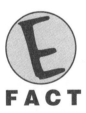

FACT

Second, third, or fourth time around? There are benefits to taking a childbirth class for even the most experienced parents. First of all, most instructors stay updated on the latest developments in obstetrical medicine, so if there's something new under the sun in labor and delivery, class is the place to learn about it. And from an altruistic viewpoint, other first-time parents will jump at the chance to hear about birth from seasoned pros. If scheduling is an issue, many facilities offer less time-intensive "brush-up" courses for veterans of the pregnancy wars.

Don't think of class as . . . well, class, either. It is an educational experience, but you aren't being graded on your performance. In other words, if academics are not your strong suit, you don't need to be in a panic. The only background you need to succeed in childbirth class is a willingness to learn and listen, and a pregnant partner. There will be no pop quizzes here.

Putting on the Coach's Hat

Coaching lesson number one: Think preschool T-ball, not major league baseball. Coaching is being supportive, helping your "rookie" learn the game of birth as she progresses through labor, giving her the tools she needs to get her through the rough spots, and above all—providing positive reinforcement and encouragement.

You likely don't need to be told this, but barking orders at your partner (assuming you would have the seriously misguided courage to do so) will get you nowhere but kicked out of the labor room. You'll learn much more about your role as coach in prepared childbirth class, but you may want to turn ahead to Chapter 18 for a preview now.

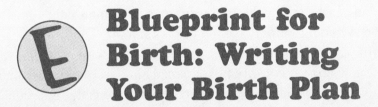

Chapter 15

Blueprint for Birth: Writing Your Birth Plan

A birth plan is a road map for your entire childbirth experience, beginning to end. It's your chance to let everyone involved (doctors, nurses, partners) know what you want the experience to be. Use it to chart the course of labor and delivery, but remember you may have to take alternate routes occasionally depending on conditions.

Why Have a Birth Plan?

The process of talking through and creating a birth plan helps you and your partner establish what you want out of childbirth (aside from the child, of course). Having it down as written word can ease your anxieties about labor and delivery. And when things get crazy as the big day arrives, a birth plan can be your calm in the storm, something solid to grasp when you suddenly seem to have forgotten just about everything you've learned.

A birth plan also serves the very important purpose of letting your provider know just what kind of experience and level of intervention you're looking for. Because it can tread on some sensitive and controversial medical territory, it's important that you include your doctor or midwife in the process.

Preparing Your Provider

Once you and your partner have your birth plan together, you should present it to your provider for his comments and questions. Communicating your wishes, and being receptive to feedback, can make the difference between a birth plan that works and one that doesn't.

Many physicians and midwives will set up a separate office visit dedicated to discussing the birth plan you've come up with. Consider the plan you take to him or her initially a "first draft." You can then incorporate your provider's input into your final plan.

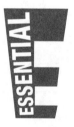

Once you have reviewed your birth plan with your practitioner, ask her to place a copy in your chart and hospital record. Make sure your labor coach and other support people who will be present at the birth have one as well so everyone is playing by the same game plan.

Unfortunately, not all practitioners are thrilled about the prospect of a birth plan. They can be a hot-button issue for some physicians who don't like to feel as if their patients don't trust them; or don't want to have a disappointed patient if the actual birth strays from the plan. For these reasons, birth plans have the potential to set up an adversarial feeling in some doctor-patient relationships.

How can you prevent your birth plan from becoming a bone of contention? First, be willing to really listen to any suggestions or issues your provider has, and make an effort to work toward a resolution together. Also, try to keep your expectations grounded in reality and not overly restrictive. Wanting your three-year-old to be nearby so she can meet her sibling shortly after birth is great, but insisting she be front and center the moment baby's head emerges is unrealistic.

Make It User-Friendly

If you hand your doctor a birth plan the size of *War and Peace*, she might start to wonder what she's gotten herself into. While covering all your bases is important, you simply can't control every possible aspect of what may, or may not, occur during labor and delivery. Medical emergencies do happen, which is why you have signed on a practitioner to begin with. You need to trust your provider to follow the *spirit* of your birth plan, while making adjustments for the health of you and your baby. Establishing a good, communicative relationship is the best way to ensure this.

Conciseness is better from a logistical viewpoint, too. The medical staff attending your birth and aftercare should be able to easily access and reference the information. Think brevity and bullet points—the Cliff's Notes of your thoughts on how you'd like birth to proceed. Keep it under five pages, if possible; fewer than that is even better.

Try to use language that is cooperative and communicative. Your birth plan should not read like a ransom note. Filling it with demands and absolutes leaves your provider very little room to make appropriate medical suggestions should birth go off-course.

The bottom line is that labor is very unpredictable and rarely do birth plans get followed to the letter. Outlining your wishes in terms of preferences, and giving your provider alternatives in case complications arise, will make your birth plan more useful to everyone involved, especially you and baby.

Atmosphere

Comfortable surroundings will help both your mind and body relax during labor. Whether you're giving birth in a hospital, at home, or somewhere in between, outlining your preference for what you'll be seeing and hearing around you is an important component of the birth plan.

The Perfect Place

First, know what you have to work with. Hospital birthing facilities are starting to recognize the value of a homey, warm atmosphere. You may find yours is already set up to suit your needs well.

However, if things look a little sterile and spartan, there are ways to make it more welcoming. Easy and acceptable additions include a cozy blanket and pillow from home, a picture or two (which serve double duty as focal points during contractions), and fresh flowers. You may also be able to adjust the lights and sounds to make things more relaxing. More on that coming up.

Home birth may also be an option if you feel strongly about giving birth in familiar surroundings and among family. However, home birth doesn't mean you should opt out of a health care professional's help; in fact, it's even more important since you won't have access to the medical monitoring and diagnostic equipment that a hospital offers. In many uncomplicated pregnancies, a home birth can be a completely safe and emotionally rewarding choice; however, women who may experience high-risk deliveries for any reason need to seriously contemplate the benefits and safety of a hospital birth.

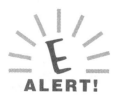

ALERT!

Be aware that professional and insurance restrictions may prohibit your doctor from attending a home birth. If your provider can't be there and your mind is set on a home birth, find out if he can refer you to a midwife or doctor who can attend.

An in-between alternative for some women might be a birthing center, which is equipped to handle some medical problems that may occur yet can offer some less conventional laboring and delivery methods such as a water birth.

Music and Lighting

Music is one of the easiest ways to change the mood. Just bring a portable stereo and a few diverse musical selections in case you need a change of pace, and you're all set. Classical music may help to soothe and center you, and something fast and furious can get the adrenaline going for the hard work. Just be conscious of the fact that other moms will likely be nearby laboring, and your baby is not wearing earplugs. Keep the volume down, or use headphones if you don't mind yet another line connecting you to something.

As far as lighting goes, you may not have a lot of choices beyond off/on if you're giving birth in a hospital setting. Even if you can dim the lights, you want your provider to be able to see what she's doing. But requesting that the drapes be drawn and the lights turned down during early and active labor is not unreasonable.

Photo Finish

Chances are you will want pictures, and lots of them. Your birth plan can outline your audiovisual expectations (e.g., video of the delivery, pictures of a C-section in the operating room, live Webcast of baby's first breath). It also serves as a good checklist for you and your partner when packing for the hospital.

If you want to capture your little star's debut on video, it's best to check with your provider to make sure there's no policy against an amateur videographer being underfoot. Even if there is, in some cases you may be able to work out a compromise, such as setting up the camera in advance on a stationary tripod.

Family, Friends, and Support

So who will be at the big event? This is perhaps one of the most crucial parts of a birth plan, to prepare for adequate support during this very difficult job that lies ahead. Is this a personal experience for just you and your partner, or do you want additional family, friends, or doula support there? It's even tougher for first-time moms, who may have misconceptions about exactly what will happen and who will be there when they hit the maternity ward.

Many women think that their provider or, at the least, a dedicated staff nurse, will be available to assist them with the entire labor and birth. In most places, that simply isn't true for a variety of reasons. Shift changes, the number of patients in labor, and other factors may have you and your partner spending a lot of time alone. Having a doula on your labor team is a great way to ensure continuity of care.

Why enlist a doula's assistance if a dad or coach is present? Many doulas will provide early labor support at home, a benefit that most practitioners can't match. It's also reassuring to many dads to know that they have a backup, and aren't forced to remember everything they learned in their 6-week childbirth class during this emotionally charged time.

If you will have people waiting at the hospital who won't be participating in your birth but who you would like to introduce to the baby as soon after as possible, indicate your wishes in the birth plan. And don't forget about a caregiver for any other, younger children who will need supervision and support.

Getting Ready

You have the people and the place set. Now for some decisions that will affect your comfort and mobility during labor.

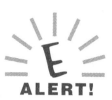

ALERT!

If you are giving birth at a hospital or other facility that allows preregistration, now is a good time to get the paperwork in order and out of the way. Preregistration allows you to file your insurance information and other necessary details with the hospital ahead of time so when labor hits you can head straight for the maternity floor, or at least check in with minimal delay.

Labor Prep Preferences

Shaving, enemas, and intravenous lines are just a few of the ways the nursing staff may get you ready for the rest of your labor and for delivery. You may have the option of doing some of these steps yourself, and forgoing others completely. Whatever you decide, make it a part of your birth plan. See Chapter 18 for more on prepping for labor.

Food and Drink

Some hospitals and providers put a strict ban on lunching during labor for several reasons. First, if things don't go as planned and you end up having a general anesthetic for a C-section, having food in your stomach puts you at risk for aspiration (inhaling vomit). Second, your stomach and gastrointestinal tract will have to digest that food when clearly there is more important action happening right next door.

That said, labor is a marathon that lasts exceedingly long for many women, who may need some sustenance to make it through. Simple, liquid-based carbohydrates such as a glass of juice, popsicle or juice bar, broth, or tea or lemonade with honey are easily digested and may give you the boost you need. Outline what you'd like to have access to so you can discuss it with your doctor. If your provider or hospital believes a light snack of food and drink is an absolute no-no in labor, intravenous lines will probably be used to take care of any risk of dehydration. However, a dry mouth is annoying and uncomfortable, so see if you can at least get ice chips to suck on and bring your lip balm.

Monitors and Mobility

Being tethered to a bed can make handling contractions and labor difficult. Yet checking the fetal heart rate and your contractions is important to ensure baby isn't encountering any stress. To give yourself room to move through the contractions while ensuring your little one's safety, ask for intermittent monitoring. Unless you require internal monitoring, which is sometimes the case in higher-risk pregnancies, having the freedom to move at least part of the time shouldn't be an issue. Newer wireless fetal monitors may let you cut the cord altogether; ask your hospital or birthing center if they use them.

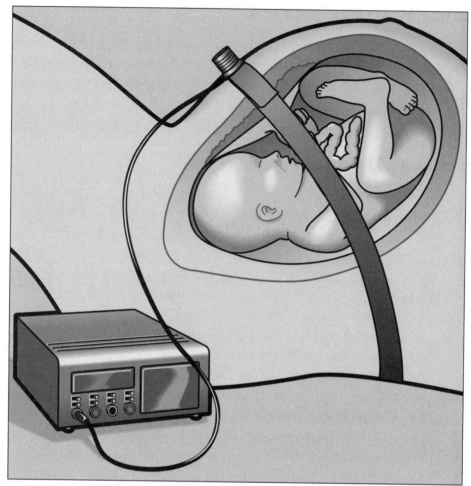

▲ A fetal monitor can assess your baby's heart rate and check for signs of fetal distress.

Pain Relief

One of the biggest decisions of childbirth is whether you will want, or need, pharmaceutical pain relief. Chapter 18 has a full assessment of your labor and delivery pain relief options. Your provider and anesthesiologist can also shed more light on the use of painkillers if you have additional questions.

Going Natural

If you intend to go completely drug-free, this section of your birth plan may be a bit more detailed than others. You'll want to outline the access you'd like to other, drug-free pain relief strategies. Things like hydrotherapy (shower or whirlpool), massage, and birth balls may be on your list. Requesting to "go natural" doesn't close the door on changing your mind. If you're a first-time mom, you can't predict whether or not pain medication will be necessary.

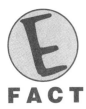

FACT

A birth ball is a large, inflatable heavy-gauge rubber ball that you can sit on, drape yourself over, or do just about anything else with that feels comfortable during a contraction. They are available in different sizes and some even come in oblong or ridged versions if you're concerned about tipping over. When used in the sitting position, the natural "give" of the ball may encourage perineal relaxation.

Timing of Pain Relief

Some practitioners may have policies about how late, or how early, in labor they will permit an epidural. Whether their policy is grounded in research, experience, or preference will probably make the difference in whether your provider is willing to be flexible on this point. If you have strong feelings about when you want access to an epidural or other pain relief option, outline your wishes in your birth plan.

When to Change Course: Interventions

Your doctor will warn you up front that unforeseen circumstances may mean a deviation from your birth plan. Sometimes women feel as if they have failed if things do not go precisely according to their concept of "the ideal birth"—which is certainly not the case. The best way to avoid disappointment is to build alternative scenarios into your birth plan regarding interventions that might be required. For example, if you really don't want an episiotomy, you should indicate that in your birth plan, and suggest perineal massage with vitamin E oil or another lubricant, warm compresses, or another acceptable alternative. But be prepared to work with your doctor during labor if your alternative plan just doesn't do the trick. And don't be too prescriptive—when you start instructing your physician in the type of sutures to use, you're forgetting that you've hired him because of his medical expertise, not in spite of it.

Some possible interventions that may come up in labor and delivery include:

- Induction
- Forceps use
- Vacuum extraction

- Episiotomy
- Artificial membrane rupture
- Labor augmentation (via the drug oxytocin, or Pitocin)

Other Considerations

The choices continue after labor and delivery, and include decisions not just about your care, but also about the care of your new son or daughter.

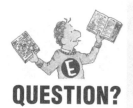

QUESTION?

I'm having a C-section. Why bother with a birth plan?
As you can see, a birth plan encompasses much more than baby's passage from point A to point B. Even with a caesarean birth, there are many choices along the way. For example, will dad be in the delivery room? Does he want to cut the cord? Can video be taken? Will you get to spend time with your baby right after the procedure? Because things can be a little more rigid rule-wise in the environment of an operating room, these are important issues to clear with your doctor ahead of time. A birth plan will help you do just that.

Cutting the Cord

You or your partner will probably be given the option to cut the baby's umbilical cord if you want to. Keep in mind that if your baby needs immediate medical attention at birth, it's possible the cord will be cut swiftly by the attending doctor or midwife instead.

The issue of when exactly to cut the cord may require some negotiations if you have strong feelings about delaying it. If your provider disagrees and believes a swift snip is in order, find out the reasons and research behind his opinion so you can explore the issue further and come to a meeting of the minds, if possible. For more on cutting the umbilical cord, see Chapter 18.

First Contact

Every woman wants her first encounter with her baby to be just perfect. After all, you've had a 9-month buildup to this moment, so wanting to stage and execute it seamlessly is natural.

If you're giving birth in a hospital, find out if there are strict procedures that must be followed with the baby's care immediately following the birth. Will you be able to nuzzle with her for as long as you'd like, or will she be whisked away for cleaning, fingerprinting, and the rest after a quick hello? Will your other children be able to meet her immediately, or will they have to wait until visiting hours? Contact your birth facility before you create this part of your plan so you aren't in for an immediate letdown if your wishes for the first meeting are against hospital policy. If you find the policies are just too restrictive, you still have time to explore other options for where you deliver.

Creative thinking may be required to make some rules and regulations acceptable to you. If you can only hold your baby for a few minutes before she goes for her after-birth tune-up, perhaps your partner can assist with those duties and use this special time to bond with baby himself.

Rooming In or Out

Do you want baby to spend just about every waking moment within arm's reach, or do you need some time to catch up on your vast sleep deficit? If it's the former, having baby spend days and particularly nights in your room with you, a setup called "rooming in," should be included in your birth plan.

Again, how much time baby sleeps with you or in the nursery may be a matter of hospital policy. However, given what research has uncovered about the importance of early bonding and nurturing and the emphasis on establishing milk supply for breastfeeding moms, it's fairly uncommon to find a facility that won't give you the choice of having your baby in the room with you. In general, you should be able to have your little one with you as much as you'd like. And if you need a short nap and the baby is not tired, the nursing staff is always there as backup.

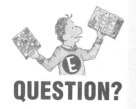

QUESTION?

I don't want my baby getting a bottle or pacifier in the hospital. Is it bad form to be so picky in the birth plan?
Not at all. It's actually helpful information to include. While your nurse will probably ask you about your feeding preferences, having it in the chart makes it easier for all involved. If you're planning on breastfeeding and want to ensure that your baby and you establish both a good technique and milk flow in those early days, it's a good idea.

Postpartum Planning

Adding a postpartum section to your birth plan can be tremendous help in getting organized after you and your baby are back at home. Will you have live-in help for a few days or weeks? Are you and your partner both taking time off? Will baby have a whirlwind schedule of introductions to friends and family, or just a few exclusive engagements?

Outline your maternity leave timetable, if you know what it is, and tentative plans for after it's over. Include baby's 2-week doctor's visit, so you won't forget to schedule it when he arrives.

Even though your health care provider won't need to put his stamp of approval on this portion of your plans, it's a good idea to run them by him. He can give you feedback on whether you'll be physically capable of doing what you've set out to do to ensure that you have a sufficient recovery period.

Appendix B in the back of this book includes a checklist you can use for guidance in creating your birth plan. (E)

Chapter 16
Month 8

Y ou are a pregnancy pro now, deftly handling all the aches and pains that come with the territory. Even if you've sailed through pregnancy feeling just fine, you've learned to adjust to the fashion hardships, the lifestyle changes, and the logistical challenges that your baby and belly have brought to the forefront. It's not much longer now.

Baby This Month

Gradually shifting to the same position in which 95 percent of all babies are born, your fetus starts to move into a head down pose, known as the vertex position. The small but stubborn percentage that don't assume the vertex position are considered breech. Feel a lot of kicking on your pelvic floor? It may be a clue that baby is still standing, or sitting, tall. She may also be lounging in the transverse position, or sideways in the womb.

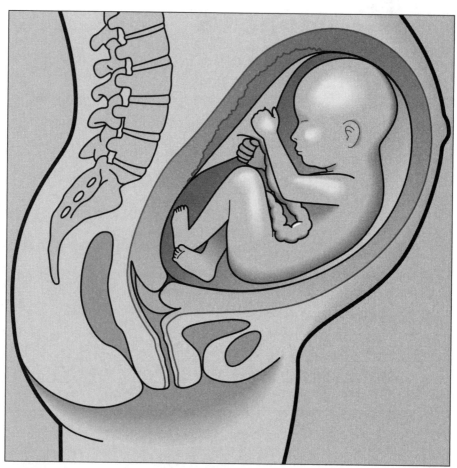

▲ You and your baby in month 8 of gestation.

Your little girl or boy is now up to 18 inches long and as heavy as a 5-pound sack of flour. The rest of her body is finally catching up to the size of her head. Although it may feel like she's constantly up and about, she's actually sleeping 90 to 95 percent of the day, a figure that will drop only slightly when she is born.

If your child were born today, she'd have an excellent chance of surviving and eventually thriving outside the womb. However, she'd still be considered preterm or premature, just as any birth before 37 weeks of gestation.

Your Body This Month

Can you still remember your prepregnancy body? The little things—like being able to zip up your coat, wear your rings, and sit on the floor without requiring adult assistance to stand again—may be a distant memory. You will not be pregnant forever, of course, although it may sometimes feel like it.

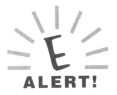

ALERT!

If you've been dribbling urine just about every time you sneeze, you're probably experiencing stress incontinence. But if you have a steady leak that seems to be unrelated to bodily stress, it may be amniotic fluid. Amniotic fluid is clear to straw-colored and has a faintly sweet smell. Less commonly, it may be tinged green or brown. If you think you're leaking amniotic fluid, no matter how small the amount, contact your care provider. If your membranes have ruptured, you risk infection if you don't deliver soon.

Your Body Changes

Weight gain should start to slow down this month. If it doesn't, however, don't cut your calorie intake below 2,600 to try and stop it. You need the extra energy for both of you.

As baby settles firmly on your bladder, bathroom stops step up once again. You may even experience some stress incontinence, which is minor dribbling or leakage of urine when you sneeze, cough, laugh, or make other sudden movements. This will clear up postpartum. In the meantime, keep doing your Kegels (see Chapter 8); don't hold it in, and wear a pantyliner.

What You Feel Like

Your Weeble-like physique has you off-balance and generally klutzy. Be careful—you wobble and you *can* fall down. And, of course, those (say it together, everyone) pregnancy hormones have loosened up your joints and relaxed your muscles to make you a bit of a butterfingers.

Now is not the ideal time to be fitted for new contacts or glasses. Pregnancy-related fluid retention can actually change the shape of your eyes and trigger minor vision changes. Also at work is estrogen, which causes your eyes to be drier than normal and may make contact lenses uncomfortable right now. Unless you want to invest in new eyewear yet again postpartum, you may want to hold off for now.

It's easier and easier to get winded as your little one pushes up into your diaphragm. Take it slow, breathe deeply, and practice good posture. To ease breathing while you sleep, pile on a few extra pillows or use a foam bed wedge to elevate your head.

Other symptoms that may continue this month include:

- Fatigue
- Frequent urination
- Tender and/or swollen breasts
- Colostrum discharge from nipples
- Bleeding gums
- Excess mucus and saliva
- Increase in normal vaginal discharge
- Mild shortness of breath
- Lightheadedness or dizziness
- Headaches
- Forgetfulness
- Gas, heartburn, and/or constipation
- Skin and hair changes
- Round ligament pain or soreness
- Lower back aches
- Mild swelling of legs, feet, and hands
- Leg cramps
- Painless, irregular contractions (Braxton-Hicks)

If you experience blurry vision or visual disturbances (e.g., spots) and you have high blood pressure or diabetes, let your provider know immediately. It could be a sign of poor control in both cases, which is dangerous to both you and your child.

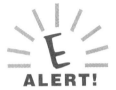

ALERT!

Although you may not relish the thought of air travel in your current wide-body state, if you do have to travel now and you aren't at risk for complications, the ACOG says it's safe to fly up through week 36. Women with placental abnormalities, pregnancy-induced hypertension, poorly controlled diabetes, sickle cell disease, or who are at risk for premature labor should remain grounded, however. If you do fly while pregnant, wear support stockings, frequently move your lower legs to prevent blood clots, and stay well hydrated.

At the Doctor

You'll see your provider twice this month as you continue your every-other-week routine. She will check the position of your baby to determine if he has turned head down in preparation for birth.

If your practitioner brings up the possibility of a breech (bottom or foot-first) birth, it's because she or he has felt the head of your unborn baby up near your ribs, or an ultrasound has confirmed that your child is in the breech position. Don't panic. Your fickle fetus is likely to change position again in the next few weeks. If she doesn't, your practitioner may try to turn the baby closer to term using a technique known as external cephalic version, or manually attempting to turn the fetus in the uterus. The ACOG recommends that an external cephalic version be attempted in most breech cases.

Babies can be delivered vaginally in breech position in some instances, but the procedure is more difficult and carries a higher risk for the infant. It is also not advised for first pregnancies. C-section is the method of choice for safe breech delivery. If you really want a vaginal birth and a cephalic version is unsuccessful in turning your breech, some practitioners may agree to a trial of labor to see if your contracting uterus helps to turn the child.

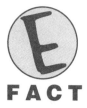

External cephalic version (or simply "version") is successful in turning a breech baby in about half of all instances where it is attempted. However, if it is done too far before the estimated delivery date, there is a possibility that the fetus may flip back to the breech position.

There are three classifications of breech: frank, complete, and incomplete. In frank breech, your baby uses your pelvic bone as a seat, and stretches his legs up close to his chest. With incomplete breech, one or both legs will drop down during delivery and will arrive before the rest of the body. This is also called a single- or double-footling breech birth. In a complete breech, your baby has his bottom on your pelvis again, but legs and arms are crossed in front of his little body.

Frank

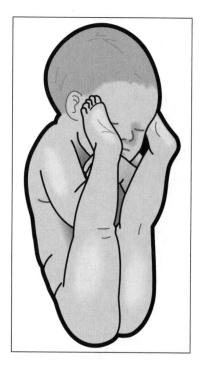

◀ There are three classifications of breech: frank, complete, and incomplete.

Complete (left) and Incomplete (right)

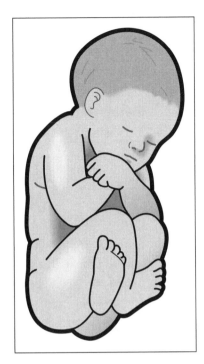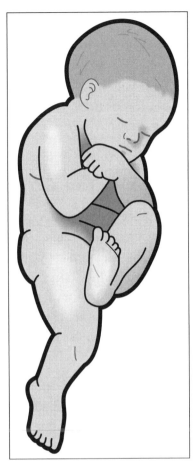

On Your Mind

As labor looms closer your thoughts turn to the task at hand. Going into labor and delivery with as much knowledge of the process as possible can make the difference between a positive childbirth experience and a long and arduous one.

Am I Up to the Task of Labor?

Women have been doing this since the beginning of time, and under much more difficult circumstances. Yes, in most cases labor will be hard work, but if you prepare yourself by learning what to expect, you will be ready to face whatever comes your way. You'll also find that your spouse or labor partner will be a huge asset in helping you through childbirth.

Am I Up to the Task of Motherhood?

In a word—yes. Great mommies are made, not born. While some parts of mothering will seem to come to you instinctively, practice and trial and error will make up the better part of your parenting education. Use the tools around you—your pediatrician, other mothers, and research and reading—to build and sharpen your skills, but listen to your inner voice in the final analysis and application of what you learn.

Things That Make You Go Grrrrr

As pregnancy winds down, your patience goes with it. The belly touchers, advice givers, urban-legend spreaders, and comedians seem to be everywhere and completely unaware of the dangerously thin ice they are treading on. Rather than biting heads off, take a deep, deep breath and remind yourself that though insensitive, most are well meaning. In the meantime, photocopy this list of no-no's for your coworkers and hang it in the break room—maybe it will sink in.

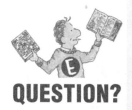

QUESTION?

What if I don't get to the hospital in time?
Every woman has heard stories of impatient babies being born in taxicabs, but these are the exception rather than the rule. Most women have plenty of time to make it to the hospital safe and sound; the average labor period runs 12 to 14 hours. But if you're concerned, you can take some basic precautions. Work out a route in advance, keep your gas tank full, and have cash on hand for a cab just in case your car decides to conk out with the first contraction.

Top 10 things not to say to a pregnant woman:

1. Haven't you had that baby yet?
2. Are you still here?
3. Wow, you're HUGE!
4. You really should avoid pain medication when you go into labor—it will hurt the baby.

5. Labor is hell! Take all the drugs you can get!
6. So how much weight have you gained?
7. You don't mind if we call you at home while you're on maternity leave, do you?
8. Are you having twins?
9. You look terrible—why don't you take a nap?
10. This is your captain speaking. Looks like our takeoff has been set back another hour. Please be aware that while we are taxiing, leaving your seat to visit the lavatory is a federal offense.

Nesting

Ahhh nesting—that overwhelming urge to turn everything in your house upside down and rearrange it just so. Your mad dash to finish the nursery and squirrel away a year's supply of diaper wipes is an instinctive reaction to baby's upcoming arrival. You're preparing a safe haven for your little one and assuring yourself that all his needs and wants will be adequately met.

A Space for Baby the First Few Weeks

Keeping baby within arm's length during her first few weeks home will improve your rest and peace of mind. A bassinet, which is about the size and depth of a baby carriage or pram, may make her feel safer and more secure than the openness of a crib. You can roll it right next to your bed and give those 4 A.M. feedings with ease. It's also an inexpensive way to bunk her down if you're still saving your pennies for the perfect crib.

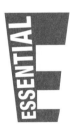

Your rest will continue to be a priority once baby arrives. If you find that having him next to your bed has you sleeping fitfully and waking up at the slightest sigh or kick, consider changing your sleeping arrangements. Have a baby monitor as backup (you'll need one anyway) just in case you find you need to keep him in his own room so both of you can get adequate sleep.

Stocking Up on Essentials

Don't go crazy buying supersized cases of baby supplies. You may not like the brand or configuration you purchase, which leaves you with a lot of unwanted merchandise on your hands. Instead, buy small so you can sample. Once you've decided what works best for you and baby, you can stock up at the warehouse store.

Some baby essentials you should have on the shelves prior to her arrival: diapers (of course), wipes, alcohol swabs (for her umbilical cord), baby shampoo and soap, diaper rash ointment, waterproof pads (a huge plus for cutting down on laundry), bottles (even if you're breastfeeding you may pump milk occasionally), a thermometer, and infant Tylenol or another fever-reducing product as recommended by your pediatrician.

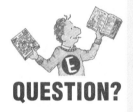

QUESTION?

What are the pros and cons of using cloth diapers?
If you're thinking green, cloth diapers have the advantage of not ending up in a landfill, although they do require additional fossil fuels and water resources to wash and transport (if you use a service). Cost can be an advantage, but it's probably a slight one if you use a service. Call local diaper services to get estimates and a run-down of what's included. You can wash them at home, of course, but be sure you have the time and the strength to be doing laundry daily. If your baby has sensitive skin, you might find cloth less irritating. Like most things in parenting, it's trial and error—have a supply of both and see how they work for you.

Just for Dads

Indecision and insecurities may plague you this month as the birth draws nearer, made all the more disturbing by your unfamiliarity with these feelings. Try to conquer your anxieties by accepting your weaknesses and valuing your strengths. And recognize the fact that learning is all part of the experience.

Measuring Up

Whether you aspire to be just like your father, or have sworn to be nothing like him at all, you've got some preconceived notion of just what makes the world's best dad. Beyond your own childhood, your idea of fatherhood has been shaped by many different influences, not the least of which are the impossibly patient patriarchs dramatized on the small screen. But while they're nice to visit, you wouldn't want to live with them. Don't try to measure up to a fantasy figure.

Start with the basics. Promise yourself you'll listen to your child, be there for him, and instill a sense of values and moral compass through your actions and your words. Love him. That's what a father does best.

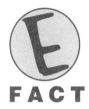

FACT

Trying to break the baby name stalemate? If you are set on one name and she on another, consider combinations of the two, or variations with first and middle. Still not agreeing? If you don't want resentments on either side, start from scratch and come up with something new that you both like. Draw on your family tree, ethnic heritage, religious beliefs, heroes and heroines, passions and hobbies, and anything else important in your life. Just make sure you consider all possible nicknames, initials, and obvious rhyming combinations to spare your child grief later.

Diaper Duty and Other Special Skills

If you're a complete novice at infant care, the best way to pick up pointers is to take a baby care class at your local hospital. You may feel silly playing with dolls at first, but when you do it in a room full of other grown men following suit, it's easier to take. However, if a class isn't an option for you, and you don't have any babies of family or friends that you can take for a test-drive, it won't take you long to learn once your baby arrives.

You'll have the opportunity to diaper your newborn during her stay in the hospital, under the watchful eye of a nurse if you so desire. This is a safe environment in which to learn if you're a little wary of your abilities.

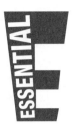

Always have a clean diaper ready and in hand before removing the soiled one. This is especially important if you have a boy. The phrase that pays: cover that guy, or get a squirt in the eye. If that doesn't help you remember, the first direct hit will. If you're diapering a girl, slide the clean diaper under her as soon as possible after the dirty one is removed (unlike a boy, you probably won't notice the puddle until it's too late). If you have a busybody that likes to get his hands into everything (including his diaper), try giving him a small toy to play with while you do your stuff.

The first bath is always cause for some jitters, but your newborn won't be having anything beyond a sponging off until she's back at home and her cord has fallen off (yes, it's supposed to do that). Tag teaming with your partner on the baby bathing is a great approach to take until you've built up your confidence level.

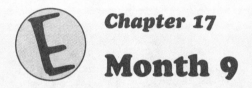

Chapter 17

Month 9

The grand finale is approaching. You may feel like you've been waiting forever. But even if you had the time of conception pinpointed, your baby may decide he needs a little more, or a little less, time preparing. Never fear—he or she will arrive sooner or later.

Baby This Month

Your child is packing on about ½ pound per week as he prepares to make his big exit. At delivery, the average U.S. birth weight is between 3,000 and 3,499 grams (6 pounds, 10 ounces, to 7 pounds, 11 ounces).

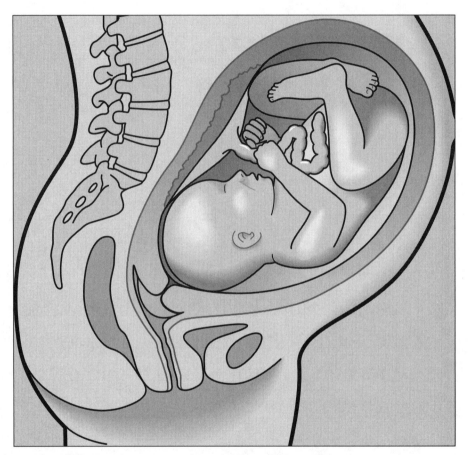

▲ A final look at you and your fetus before the big day.

He's fully formed and just waiting for the right time now. If you're having a boy, his testicles have descended and may be visible in any 9-month ultrasound images. His lungs, the last organ system to fully mature, now have an adequate level of surfactant in them to allow breathing outside of the womb.

A dark, tarry amalgam of amniotic fluid, skin cells, and other fetal waste, is gathering in your baby's intestines. This substance, called meconium, will become the contents of his bowel movements during the first few days of life.

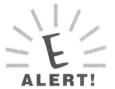

ALERT!

Fetal movement will naturally become less vigorous as you get closer to your due date and the baby is pressed for space, but a healthy baby should still be making his presence known. Your provider may ask you to count fetal kicks. Pick a typically active time of day for your little one and start counting his moves. Your provider will let you know how many movements you should feel in what period of time (usually around 8 to 10 in a space of 2 hours). If she seems slow, she may be sleeping. Try drinking a glass of juice to get her going. Call your provider immediately if baby's movements are notably decreased or absent.

Your Body This Month

While baby is still growing, your weight gain tapers off and you may even lose 1 pound or so due to a drop in amniotic fluid production. Groin soreness and backaches are more persistent as the musculoskeletal system strains to support your abdomen. The good news—you can't get any bigger.

Your Body Changes

Engagement or lightening, the process of the baby "dropping" down into the pelvic cavity in preparation for delivery, may occur any time now. In some women (particularly those who have given birth before), it may not happen until labor starts.

Your cervix is ripening (softening) in preparation for baby's passage. As it effaces (thins) and dilates (opens), the soft plug of mucus keeping it sealed tight may be dislodged. This mass, which has the appealing name of mucus plug, may be tinged red or pink, and is also referred to as the equally explicit bloody show.

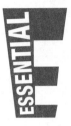

A pregnancy is considered full-term from 37 to 42 weeks. Only 5 percent of expectant women actually give birth on their estimated date of delivery, and first-time moms are more likely to go past their due date. If you've delivered a baby before, however, you are more likely to give birth within 4 days of your EDD.

What You Feel Like

If the baby has dropped, you may be running to the bathroom more than ever. He also may be sending shockwaves through your pelvis as he settles further down onto the pelvic floor. On the upside, you can finally breathe as he pulls away from your lungs and diaphragm. Braxton-Hicks contractions may be more frequent this month as you draw nearer to delivery. You're close enough to be on the lookout for the real thing, however. How will you recognize them?

Real contractions will:

- Be felt in the back and possibly radiate around to the abdomen.
- *Not* subside when you move around or change positions.
- Increase in intensity as time passes.
- Come at roughly regular intervals (early on this may be from 20 to 45 minutes apart).
- Increase in intensity with activity like walking.

Other signs that labor is on its way include amniotic fluid leaks in either a gush or a trickle (your "water breaking"), sudden diarrhea, and the appearance of the mucus plug. Keep in mind, however, that for many women, the bag of waters does not break until active labor sets in.

At the Doctor

You'll see your doctor on a weekly basis now until you deliver. Unless you are scheduled for a planned caesarean, your provider will probably perform an internal exam with each visit to check your cervix for changes that indicate approaching labor.

Tests This Month

The U.S. Centers for Disease Control recommends that your provider administer a group B strep (GBS) test one month prior to your estimated delivery date. This culture is performed by swabbing a fluid sample from both your vagina and rectum. If the cultured fluid comes back positive for GBS, you may have antibiotics administered during delivery to prevent transmission to the baby.

Checking Your Cervix

Your provider will be checking your cervix for signs that it is preparing for your baby's passage. She'll also be taking note of any descent or dropping of the baby toward the pelvis, called the station. Take the numbers you hear with a grain of salt, however. Although you may start effacing and dilating now, it's still anyone's guess as to when labor will begin, and it could be a few more weeks yet.

On Your Mind

You're likely tired but happy as you pack and prepare for the big day. Just remember the "estimated" in estimated delivery date to avoid a big letdown if baby is tardy.

Tired of Being Pregnant

You are *so* ready to have this baby. Nothing fits, not even your shoes. You can't sleep for more than a few hours at a time. Your belly itches and your breasts ache. You look toward your due date like a long distance runner approaching the end of a marathon. As you waddle toward the finish line, enjoy these final sensations of your child moving inside of you—the funny little hiccups, the elbow and knee bumps parading across your belly, and the subtle nudges that remind you you're not alone even if no one else is around.

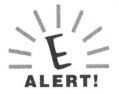

ALERT!

When your cervix hasn't budged and your due date has come and gone, you may be tempted to try one of those surefire homemade labor inducers that every pregnant woman hears about. Castor oil, herbal concoctions, spicy food, and sex are just a few methods bandied about in pregnancy chat rooms everywhere. Unfortunately, some may only succeed in making you nauseous, while others may pose a real danger. Even if you're embarrassed, you need to run it by your doctor or midwife before taking matters into your own hands. A good provider will listen, and won't laugh, letting you know what's safe and what isn't.

Irritable and Anxious

As sleep gets more and more elusive and your discomfort level ratchets up, you may find yourself easily provoked. The best short-term solution to keeping your cool? Stay clear of encounters with people you just know will irritate you (whether they mean to or not), and ask your significant other to be the point person on all "anything yet?" questions.

First-time moms may find themselves overwhelmed with anxiety now that birth is so near. Take a deep breath, go over what you learned in childbirth class (repeatedly if it helps ease your mind), and talk with your partner or labor coach about ways to relax and get past the anxious feelings. It's perfectly natural to be fearful of the unknown, but don't let fear wrest control of your labor from you.

Even if you have been through pregnancy already, you may still be anxious about baby's arrival. Perhaps you're following a different kind of labor and birth plan, or you're concerned about how your other child will react to his new brother or sister. Again, talk it out with your partner, ask your provider any questions that may still be on your mind about labor and delivery, and remember that you've been through this once and you'll make it through again.

Excited and Happy

How could you not be excited? You're finally going to meet the little one you've known only through kicks, hiccups, and grainy ultrasound images. Will she look like you? What will you do when you get to hold her for the first time? Relish these final days of exhilaration and anticipation—they are truly unique.

Gearing Up for the Big Event

Since baby's timetable is somewhat unpredictable, start getting your affairs in order at the beginning of this month. Cover all personal, professional, and family bases to ensure a smooth transition from home to hospital and back home again.

Finalize the Birth Plan

Double-check with your provider that a copy of your birth plan has been put into your chart, and verify any changes you might have made to the plan since your first review together. Provide your labor coach with an extra copy just in case the original is misplaced.

Pack Your Bag

You'll probably pack and unpack your bag a half dozen times this month making sure you have everything you could possibly need. Don't go crazy with books, notebook computers, or other work or entertainment equipment. You'll be too busy with labor, delivery, and the blissful preoccupation of meeting and caring for your child.

Essentials you should have:

- **Pain-relief tools for labor.** Things like massage balls, a picture for focusing on through contractions, a water bottle, and so forth.
- **Music to labor by.** Check with your hospital or birthing center in advance to see if a small portable stereo is acceptable. If not, you can always bring personal headphones.
- **Snacks for the coach.** Make sure it's something that won't turn your stomach if you see or smell it during labor.
- **A camera.** For capturing baby's arrival (or the moments shortly thereafter). Don't forget the batteries and film (or an extra memory card)!

- **Stopwatch, clock, or watch with a second hand.** For timing contractions.
- **Several nightgowns.** With button or snap fronts if you're going to nurse.
- **Extra underwear.** Make them comfortable but not your best—they'll probably end up with some postpartum bloodstains.
- **Sanitary pads.** The hospital will provide you with some, but extras are good to have on hand.
- **Phone numbers.** Make sure your partner has names and numbers of the folks you'll want to clue in immediately on the new arrival.
- **A small gift from baby to any siblings.** A "hello big sister/brother" gift can make their introduction smoother.
- **A picture of the kids.** Taping a picture of big brother or sister to your newborn's bassinet is a good way to emphasize your first child's important new role in the family.
- **Glasses or contacts.** Make sure you can see the baby after he's finally here.
- **Warm socks and/or slippers.** Those hospital floors can be cold.
- **A bathrobe.** For hallway walks to the nursery.
- **A baby blanket.** For baby's return home. Let your partner bring the car seat on discharge day so you aren't overwhelmed with luggage.
- **Toiletries.** Toothbrush, toothpaste, and other basics.
- **Shower supplies.** You'll be given an opportunity to shower at the hospital, so pack shampoo and other necessities.
- **A going-home outfit for both you and baby.** Pack a set of newborn clothes, and make sure you bring something loose and comfortable to wear yourself.

If you're breastfeeding, you might also pack:

- **Nursing bras.** If you don't have any yet, a bra with a front fastener will work well as a stand-in for now.
- **A box of nursing pads.** For when your milk comes in.
- **Vitamin E oil or lanolin ointment.** For sore or cracked nipples.

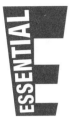

Don't put your prepregnancy jeans in your hospital bag. You're sure to be sorely disappointed. While you'll lose a large percentage of the weight you've gained this past 9 months, it will take some time to return to your old shape and size. If the thought of putting on maternity clothes yet again postpartum is too depressing, buy a comfortable but stretchy "coming-home" outfit in a new-mom-friendly size.

Recruit Help Now!

Now is the time to take up friends, family, and neighbors on their offers of assistance.

If they ask if they can help, by all means, take them up on it. Make a list and schedule assignments. Give friends that are good in the kitchen cooking detail, so you can have a supply of frozen, home-cooked meals on hand for easy dinners. If you have other children, charge your husband or partner with making sure their school, extracurricular, and social schedules are covered.

Feel like you need some live-in help to get you through the first week or so? Ask a mommy-expert, maybe even your own mom, to come for a visit. Sound out the idea with your mate; he may feel this is a special "just the three of you" family time, but also might reconsider if he hears your reasons. Just make sure your guest isn't someone who will be driving you bonkers after 2 days.

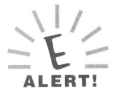

Having a cesarean section? You'll be recovering from major surgery as well as going through new-mom adjustments. It's essential you have adequate rest and support so you can heal and care for baby. Federal law mandates that your health insurer must cover at least 4 days of hospitalization following an uncomplicated C-section birth. If your insurance covers more and your provider gives you a choice, stay as long as you can.

Finalize Maternity Leave Plans

If you're working right up until your due date, start clearing the decks early in the month. Make sure coworkers and managers are regularly apprised of where outstanding projects stand, and try to treat every day as if it may be your last before leave. The more you enable things to flow smoothly in your absence, the less likely you are to get calls at home.

Talk with your supervisor about communication in your absence. If you want to remain incommunicado (and you have every right to do so), make your feelings known. You might think about setting a limit on any contact you do agree to, such as e-mails only, which may be easier to answer at your leisure when baby is asleep, or phone calls only in a certain window of time each day. Be sure to outline circumstances that you would consider important enough to be disturbed for. Remember—this is your time off to both recuperate and get to know your child. Your workplace will survive. For more on working through pregnancy and beyond, see Chapter 9.

Hurry Up and Wait (When Baby Is Late)

You've finally reached that magic EDD number and . . . nothing. No fanfare, no contractions, and definitely no baby. Disappointed, you resign yourself to yet another day of pregnancy. Don't be too depressed. Instead, try to stay busy and if you feel up to it, get out and about. A nice long walk may be just what your little one needs for inspiration. Sitting at home, analyzing every twitch of your abdomen, and watching the hours crawl by will only make the waiting longer.

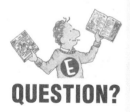

QUESTION?

I'm 1 week overdue. Will my provider induce me if I request it?
Whether or not to induce depends on a number of factors. Is the cervix effaced or dilated? Are you fairly sure your due date was accurate to begin with? Have you had a previous C-section? Generally speaking, if you've hit the 41-week mark, you have no history of C-section, and your provider thinks induction is indicated, she will schedule one for you. For more on induction, page ahead to Chapter 18.

Unless you have a precise 28-day cycle and are positive of the exact day that sperm met egg, gestational dating can be fuzzy at best. If you are 1 week or more past the EDD, your provider will order additional tests, including a biophysical profile, which includes a non-stress test (NST) and ultrasound assessment of amniotic fluid levels and fetal size. These tools will give her a much better picture of whether or not baby is ready to arrive.

Babies who stay in the womb 42 weeks or longer are considered post-term or postdate. Postdate pregnancies may develop macrosomia, or large body size of 4,000 grams (8 pounds, 13 ounces) or more that may make it difficult to pass through the birth canal. A postdate fetus may also pass meconium, the black tarry stool that is baby's first bowel movement. If meconium is released into the amniotic fluid, it has the potential to cause fetal distress by blocking the airway. That's why regular assessment of a post-date pregnancy is extremely important.

Just for Dads

It's showtime! Finally, you'll be able to get into the parenting act on a more hands-on level. As the baby's due date approaches, remember that your partner needs you more than ever. Spoil her a little—or even a lot.

Getting Her to the Hospital

Having nightmares about having to deliver the baby in the back seat of your Ford Taurus? Perhaps it will ease your mind to hear that the average first-time mom is in labor for about 14 hours (women in later pregnancies tend to have shorter labors—around an 8-hour average), more than enough time to get to the hospital.

Remembering everything in the thrill of the big moment may be hard, so make yourself a checklist and keep it on your dash: one overnight bag, your list of phone numbers, plenty of change for phone calls, and of course, one laboring mommy-to-be. And make a habit of topping off your tank every time it reaches the half-empty mark so you won't have to stop for gas.

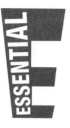

Bring your calling card or a pocketful of change for your long list of phone calls. Many hospitals do not allow cell phone use inside the building due to the risk of interference with sensitive medical equipment. Although some facilities are starting to allow less obtrusive digital wireless phones (primarily for staff communications), chances are you'll have to rely on the pay phone for now.

False Alarms

Many women hit the hospital certain that they're just hours away from birth, only to be told they're just a few centimeters dilated. There is no bigger letdown for a very pregnant woman, particularly one who is past her due date, to be sent home from the hospital with baby still on board. She may get teary, frustrated, exasperated, and convinced that she'll be pregnant forever. Even though you may be disappointed by the delay as well, give her a good shoulder to cry on and offer some extra TLC.

Running Interference

Taking over phone duty this month can help ease your partner's stress significantly. Chances are family, friends, neighbors, and anyone else who knows the big day is approaching will be calling for a status report. As the due date draws near, this can be a nuisance, but when the date has come and gone, it escalates into the unbearable zone. Let your spouse know you'll field the phone calls for now and pass along anything of consequence. If it gets to be too much of a deluge, you might gently remind your callers that they're on your list to contact once something does occur. Ⓔ

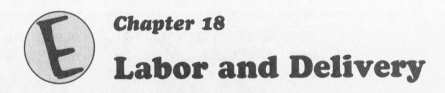

Chapter 18

Labor and Delivery

Even if you've read just about everything about labor and delivery, took copious notes in childbirth class, and questioned all your friends on their experiences, you'll still find your labor experiences different in some way from the others. Every woman's labor is unique, and so comparisons of length, progress, and pain perception can be inaccurate, or even discouraging. Follow your own path and you'll do fine.

Get Ready: Baby and Your Body in Labor

Labor is hard work (don't let anyone tell you otherwise) but it's also the most rewarding work you'll ever do.

Contractions

The first signal of labor is contractions—the tightening and release of your uterus that helps propel your baby down the birth canal. These contractions are different than the Braxton-Hicks you may have had, in that they occur at regular intervals, are painful, and are slowly but surely opening the door (i.e., cervix) for baby's exit.

You don't need to rush to the hospital or birthing center after your first contraction. But you should call your doctor or midwife and let them know labor has started and how far apart contractions are (from the beginning of one to the start of the next). Your provider will let you know at what point you should head for the hospital or birthing center. Until then, you can labor in the comfort and privacy of your own home. However, if the pain starts to be more than you can handle without professional help, call your provider back and let her know. Read on for early pain relief options you can try at home.

Prep

When you do arrive at your birthing center or hospital, the nursing staff will prep, or prepare you, for labor and delivery. What prepping involves depends on facility policy and doctor preference, but here are some procedures you may encounter.

Suit Up

You'll change into your hospital gown or gear from home. Try not to wear a lot of jewelry or other extraneous items that may get lost.

A Close Shave

Though it's not as common as it used to be, you may be getting a partial shave of your perineal area or less commonly, a full shave of both your abdominal and pubic area. The rationale is to prevent possible infection and improve visibility for your doctor.

The Enema Within

Yes, your hospital may require an enema to clear out your bowel so baby will have a smoother passage down the neighboring birth canal. Find out in advance if this is required; you may be able to administer it at home if it makes you more comfortable. If contractions have had you on the toilet all day and you've got nothing left to give, let your nurse know and they may bypass this step.

Drop a Line

Your nurse may insert a needle with a heparin lock, and secure it with surgical tape. If IV medication is suddenly needed during labor, it can be easily administered. Other hospitals will hook you up to an intravenous (IV) line as a matter of course and "feed" you a glucose solution to keep you hydrated. Again, other medications can be added to the line as necessary.

Baby Monitor

Chances are good you've experienced the fetal monitor during a visit to your provider, so this part of the procedure may be familiar to you. The monitor will give you a look at your contractions, and it will allow you and your coach to see when one is coming and more importantly, when it seems to be almost over. It will also pick up fetal heart sounds and alert you to any stress the baby may be experiencing from oxygen deprivation or problems with the umbilical cord. An internal monitor may be used if you are considered to be at high risk. For more on fetal monitoring, see Chapter 5.

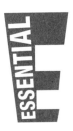

If you don't want to be chained to your bed during labor, find out if your birth facility has fetal monitors that use telemetry technology. These wireless monitors strap on like a regular external device, but you don't have to remain plugged into anything. You may have to remain in the same room with the base unit, however, depending on the type of system. There are even telemetry units that are waterproof in case a mom wants to ease labor pains with hydrotherapy.

Get Set: Pain Relief Options

In early labor, when contractions are getting intense but are still not close enough so that you should leave for the hospital, there are a few ways you can ease the pain.

Nonmedical Solutions

First, have plenty of pillows on hand. Experiment with different positions, such as on all fours, against a wall, and leaning against someone or something while bent forward at the waist.

Back labor, which occurs when baby's face is toward your abdomen rather than your spine, can cause severe lower back pain. Ask your partner to try massage or a warm water bottle to ease contractions. The soothing jets of a whirlpool tub can do wonders if you have one. However, if your water has broken, never take a soak without approval from your provider.

Keep positive, supportive people around you. Let your coach be your buffer, and clear out any distractions. Try to remain focused on riding through and past the contraction. Fix your eyes on something that relaxes you and practice the breathing exercises you learned in childbirth class to keep the oxygen and blood flowing. Don't hyperventilate. Talk or groan through the height of the contraction if it helps.

It's difficult to relax while you're in the midst of a really big, really uncomfortable contraction. However, letting go in between contractions can help ease your mind and body and loosen you up for impending delivery. You may have learned a few relaxation exercises in childbirth class. If so, now is the time to try them, as they can make the pain more manageable.

Progressive relaxation, which is a series of muscle tightening and release, is a good way to release your stress. Make sure you're in comfortable clothes in a soothing atmosphere (i.e., quiet and perhaps dim). Recline with your head and back elevated, and start tensing and then releasing each muscle group, from your head to your toes. Breathe in with the tension, and blow it out with the release. Try to clear your head of everything but the sensation at hand. If you practice this prior to labor, it can be a good tool for managing some of the early pain when contractions are still relatively far apart.

Pharmaceutical Options

Once you arrive at the hospital, you will have analgesics and anesthetics available for pain relief if you choose to have them.

Analgesics

Analgesics deaden the pain by depressing your nervous system. They make you sleepy and help you rest between contractions. The analgesics Demerol (meperidine), Stadol (butorphanol), Nubain (nalbuphine), and morphine are commonly used in labor. Although some of these drugs, such as Demerol, may even allow you to nap between contractions, you remain conscious (albeit a bit giddy) under their influence. While these medications can cross the placenta, when they are properly administered in the appropriate dosages they should not cause baby any serious side effects.

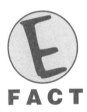

FACT

Pain relief in labor was roundly condemned for many centuries, partly on biblical grounds (think Eve and the apple), until Queen Victoria of England requested and was administered chloroform for the birth of her eighth and ninth children. The births of both Prince Leopold and Princess Beatrice were attended by Dr. John Snow, a pioneer in anesthetic use. After Prince Leopold was born in 1853, the Queen praised the relief chloroform provided, thus legitimizing the obstetrical use of anesthetic and the further advancement of the field.

General Anesthesia

You may also receive either a general or local (regional) anesthetic. A general anesthesia brings about a complete loss of consciousness, or "puts you to sleep." General anesthesia is rarely used in labor and delivery; usually only in cases of an emergency cesarean section where there isn't adequate time to prep the patient with a local anesthetic. Newborns arriving under the influence of a general anesthesia may be drowsy and slow to respond due to the effects of the anesthesia.

Local Anesthesia

Local anesthesia, also called regional anesthesia, numbs only a specific portion of the body and leaves you awake and alert. The most commonly used local anesthesia is probably the lumbar epidural. Injected into the space between two vertebrae of your lower back (the epidural space), this type of anesthesia is administered when you are well into labor and will temporarily numb the nerves all the way from your belly button to your knees. An epidural takes 20 minutes to start working and can also lower your blood pressure. For this reason, you'll be put on the fetal monitor and hooked up to an IV fluid drip if you're given an epidural.

Some providers may require you to wait until you reach a certain dilation benchmark or stage of labor to have an epidural, but if you are being induced, an epidural may be in order earlier since you may experience a lot of pain before there is any major progress in the dilatation of your cervix. Most providers will give you more time to push with an epidural because your sensation is impaired. If you have concerns about epidural timing, discuss them with your health care provider.

The epidural is administered through a small plastic catheter in your back. An anesthesiologist will place the epidural catheter and administer the local anesthetic agent. Before he starts, your lower back will be draped and the insertion spot swabbed with antiseptic or iodine. You may be asked to pull your knees and chin toward your chest so your spine is more visible. The catheter is inserted in the space between the fourth and fifth vertebrae and the anesthesia injected into it. You may feel a slight stinging sensation down your legs, but your breathing and the involuntary muscles working those contractions won't be affected. The insertion of an epidural catheter allows anesthetics to be administered on an "as needed basis" and is useful should a C-section ultimately be required.

After insertion, the doctor will secure the catheter and you can get comfortable again. Watch the fetal monitor for the start of the next contraction. You'll be amazed at how what was turning you inside out a moment ago is barely perceptible now. The numbness will take several hours to wear off and may restrict your movements during the birth, but an epidural can be a great pain management tool.

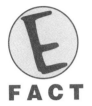

FACT

A spinal block, like an epidural, is administered in the lower back. However, a spinal is delivered directly into the fluid around your spinal cord, not into the spaces between your vertebrae as in an epidural. Used right at delivery only or during a C-section, the spinal will numb you all the way from your rib cage down.

Women who would like to have the pain relief benefits of an epidural but would also like to retain the ability to move around during labor may be candidates for a low-dose combination spinal epidural, sometimes referred to as a walking epidural. An epidural catheter is inserted, and an injection of a narcotic is administered into the spinal fluid by using a smaller needle that fits through the epidural catheter. A walking epidural is usually faster acting than a conventional epidural, and it allows you to retain enough sensation to move and walk, which can speed the labor process.

Other anesthetic blocks that are used less frequently include:

- A caudal block is administered into the bony area right at the end of your spine, and affects the abdominal and pelvic muscles.
- A saddle block is a type of low spinal that numbs a more limited area of your body—your perineum, inner thighs, and bottom.
- With a paracervical block, the anesthetic is injected into either side of your cervix during labor to numb the area.
- With a pudendal block, the anesthetic is administered to the nerves around the vagina and pelvic floor to help control pain when the baby's head bulges into your cervix.

Go! Labor in Three Acts

Labor is a series of three distinct stages, aptly called first, second, and third stages. For most women, the longest distance to cover is the first stage, which lasts from the earliest signs of labor right through baby's descent into the birth canal in preparation for stage two—pushing. Stage three consists of delivering the placenta, which some mothers feel is a cakewalk after all the hard work involved in baby's arrival.

First Stage

The first stage of labor is actually a three-part act itself, consisting of early (latent), active, and transition (descent) labor.

During the early phase, the cervix effaces (thins) and dilates (opens). This ripening process may have started several weeks ago, well before the regular contractions of early labor began (see Chapter 17). Now, your cervix will dilate to about 4 or 5 centimeters. Contractions will arrive every 15 to 20 minutes and last 60 to 90 seconds. If your partner or coach isn't around, now is the time to contact him so he can be by your side. Then touch bases with your provider, who will tell you at what point you should head to the hospital or birthing facility.

Try to stay up and moving through contractions as much as you can to let gravity help your baby descend. Consider a light liquid snack (e.g., broth or juice) to power up your energy reserves for the long road ahead. Rest if possible. Try the breathing and relaxation techniques you picked up in childbirth class, and coach-assisted massage or showering to get you through these first few hours. Then leave for the hospital and the next stage—active labor.

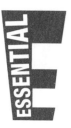

If your birthing center or hospital has whirlpool tubs or showers available for laboring moms, you may find the pulsating water welcome relief for pulling through contractions. This pain relief method—called hydrotherapy—is not the same as a water birth, in which a baby is actually born submerged in a pool of water.

In active labor, your contractions are coming closer together regularly, perhaps 3 to 5 minutes apart, and they can be intense, lasting 45 seconds. These strong contractions are dilating your cervix from about 4 to 5 centimeters to around 8 (when transition begins).

Once you reach the birthing center or hospital, you'll be quickly prepped as described earlier and given an internal exam to check the progress of your cervix. The baby's position will be checked and you will probably be hooked up to a fetal monitor to assess the baby's well-being. (See Chapter 5 for more on fetal monitoring.)

Other signs that active labor is in progress:

- Your membranes rupture. If the amniotic sac hasn't already broken, it will now or very soon.
- You bleed from your vagina. More of the mucus plug is being expelled.
- You need air. Put those cleansing breaths and other breathing techniques into practice. Your hardworking uterus needs oxygen.
- Your back *really* hurts. The baby's head is pushing on your backbone. Massage may help.
- You have muscle cramps. Again, massage may help the ill-timed charley horse.
- You're exhausted and physically spent. Remember what you're working toward. Let your coach know how you're feeling so he can motivate you and get you whatever he can to keep moving forward.

Don't feel inadequate or guilty about asking for pain medication at any point if you want and need it. You wouldn't hesitate to take novocaine if you were getting a wisdom tooth pulled, yet having an 8-pound child pulled through a 10-centimeter opening doesn't qualify? Pain medication is a tool, just like your breathing exercises. Wisely used, it can result in a better birth experience for both you and your child.

Once your cervix reaches 8 centimeters and contractions start coming one on top of another to get you to full dilation, transition has arrived. Because of the frequency of contractions and the overwhelming urge to push, this is the most difficult part of labor. Fortunately, it culminates in your child's delivery once you bridge those final 2 centimeters to being fully dilated.

During transition:

- You could be nauseous and may even vomit.
- You have the chills or sweats and your muscles twitch.
- Your back *really, really* hurts.
- Contractions are just minutes apart, if even that.
- There is pressure in your rectum from the baby.

- You are absolutely exhausted.
- You may feel like pushing even though your cervix is not yet fully dilated.

Although every fiber of your body may be screaming "PUSH!" you need to hold back just a few moments more. Your cervix is almost, but not quite, open far enough for baby's safe passage. Take quick shallow breaths and resist the urge until your doctor or midwife gives the go-ahead.

Second Stage, or PUSH!

Your cervix has made it to 10 centimeters and you are finally allowed to push. This second stage can last anywhere from a few minutes (with second or subsequent babies) to several hours. Your contractions will still arrive regularly, but they aren't quite as close together, a welcome relief. Pushing is very hard work, but the sensations may change from the intense gripping you've experienced to more of a stinging or burning sensation.

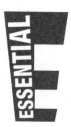

If possible, try to find a pushing position that doesn't attempt to defy gravity. Instead, use gravity to your advantage by kneeling, squatting, or sitting up with your legs and knees spread far apart. Stirrups may be available, but don't feel forced into using them if they don't work for you.

Your birth attendant and/or coach will let you know when the peak of the contraction occurs, the optimum time for pushing effectively. Use whatever it takes to push effectively. If that means moaning, grunting, and other primal sounds that make your prenatal snoring sound like a lullaby in comparison, go for it. The people attending your birth have probably seen just about everything. Don't be embarrassed, because it won't even phase them.

The emergence of the head at your vaginal opening starts with a small patch of skin visible during the peak of a push. The patch may recede when you rest but will reappear at the next contraction. Unless your baby is arriving in a breech position, the head will finally crown, or bulge right out of your vaginal opening. You may be asked to stop pushing momentarily as the baby's head is ready to emerge in order to prevent perineal tearing. Panting can help you suppress the urge. The obstetrician or midwife may decide on an episiotomy if your skin doesn't appear to be willing to stretch another millimeter, or they may attempt perineal massage.

Finally, the head slides face down past the perineum and is eased out carefully by the birth attendant to prevent injury to the baby. The attendant may wipe the eyes, nose, and mouth and suction any mucus or fluid from her upper respiratory tract. It's all downhill from here as the rest of the body slides out.

As your baby leaves the quiet, dim warmth of the womb for the bright lights and big noises of the outside world, his respiratory reflexes kick in and the newborn lungs fill with air for the first time. He'll probably test out those lungs with a full-fledged wail.

Your doctor will place the baby on your stomach for introductions, usually with the umbilical cord still attached.

The cord will continue to pulse with blood flow for a few minutes. The timing of the actual clamping and severing of the cord will depend upon your practitioner, and this is a matter of some debate in childbirth circles. Some professionals believe that waiting until pulsation has stopped, or even until after the placenta is delivered, improves baby's circulation and blood pressure and reduces mom's chance of hemorrhage. Other practitioners cite a higher incidence of jaundice in newborns with delayed cord cuts and believe in clamping and cutting earlier. You may want to talk it over with your doctor if you have concerns about the timing of the cord cut. If baby requires resuscitation, if the cord is tightly wrapped around a body part, or if it is exceedingly short, it will be cut sooner.

Most practitioners will give dad, or even mom, the option of cutting the cord in an uncomplicated birth. Don't feel bad if it isn't your cup of tea, especially if either one of you is a bit squeamish. Better to spend the time cuddling your baby than being picked up off the delivery room floor.

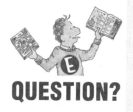

QUESTION?

What is umbilical cord banking?
The umbilical cord blood contains stem cells, those miraculous little blank slates from which all organs and tissues are built. Cord blood collected immediately after birth is placed in a collection kit and flown to a facility where it is cryogenically frozen and "banked" for later use if needed. The theory behind cord banking is that if your child ever develops a disease or condition requiring stem-cell treatment, the cord blood can be thawed and used for her treatment. If it matches certain biological markers, cord blood can be used to treat other family members as well. However, banking is cost-prohibitive for many and requires an annual storage fee for as long as you'd like to keep the cord blood frozen.

Third, or, You Aren't Done Yet

The third stage of labor is the delivery of the placenta. The entire placenta must be expelled to prevent bleeding complications later on. Contractions will continue, and your doctor may press down on your abdomen and massage your uterus, or tug gently on the end of the umbilical cord hanging from your vagina. You may also be injected with the hormone Pitocin (oxytocin) to step up your contractions and expel the placenta. You'll be given pushing directives again, but this part will seem like a piece of cake given the task you've just completed.

Once the placenta is out, any stitches you require to repair tearing or episiotomy incisions will be put in. A local anesthetic will be injected to deaden the area if you aren't still anesthetized from an epidural.

Caesarean Section

A caesarean birth may be scheduled for you if you have a breech baby or other complications or conditions that indicate the need for a C-section. It may also be performed in emergency situations where the fetus is in distress. A caesarean is major abdominal surgery and carries with it all the risks of infection and complication that any surgical procedure does. On the positive side, with a planned C-section your due date is your due date, and no contractions are necessary unless you begin to labor before the date.

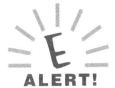

ALERT!

If you are having a scheduled caesarean, try to arrange a few moments to consult with the anesthesiologist ahead of time. If you've had any poor experiences with anesthesia in prior C-sections, let her know so you can improve the outcome this time around. She can also answer any questions you might have about her part of the procedure.

In Advance of the Surgery

If you have any advance warning about your C-section, you'll probably be offered an epidural or spinal rather than general anesthesia. Before the procedure begins, you'll be prepped. A nurse will shave the area of the incision, and your arm will be hooked up to an intravenous line to receive fluids as well as pain medication. You may also be asked to drink an antacid solution called sodium citrate to neutralize your stomach acid.

Before the procedure begins you will have a catheter inserted into your bladder. The anesthetic block will give you little control over the muscles that control urine flow, so the catheter will do the work for you both during and after the procedure. Catheter insertion can be uncomfortable, so ask that it be inserted after you've received your anesthetic block (which will likely be in the operating room).

In the Operating Room

Once you're prepped, you will be wheeled to the operating room. In the operating room, the anesthesiologist will have you roll on your side and pull your knees toward your chest, or sit with your legs dangling off the table, while he inserts a fine needle and catheter for an epidural or spinal block into your back. You'll then be asked to lay flat on your back with your arms straight out to the sides. A curtain just a few feet high will be positioned at your chest to keep the surgical field (the area where all the action is) sterile. This will also block your view of the procedure, so if you're determined to see baby the moment she emerges, you will want to ask for an appropriately placed mirror as early as possible.

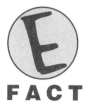

FACT

A severe headache known as postdural or post-puncture spinal headache is an uncommon but highly uncomfortable potential side effect of spinal blocks and epidurals. It is caused by the change in spinal fluid pressure that occurs if spinal fluid leaks out into the epidural space during or after the procedure. It may be more common in spinal blocks because of the larger needle size used. Rest and fluids usually resolve the problem, but in some cases an injection of blood into the epidural space, called a blood patch, may be required to seal the puncture site.

Your arms may be loosely fastened down with Velcro straps. This is not to keep you from jumping off the table, but to prevent any accidental movements that again may breach the sterility of the surgical field.

The most uncomfortable part of the C-section procedure itself is arguably the flat-on-your-back part. It's quite possible you will get nauseous as your heavy uterus compresses your vena cava and starts to lower your blood pressure. In addition, the anesthetic itself may cause your blood pressure to fall. Although the anesthesiologist will administer medication to control this drop, called hypotension, you may get sick to your stomach. Think how long you can stand laying flat on your back at 9 months pregnant, and you'll see why. The discomfort is compounded by the fact that, if necessary, you will have to vomit laying down with your head turned to the side. This is where a well-placed mate, tray in hand, is indispensable. If this does happen, just remember it will likely be short-lived.

The obstetrician will make an incision, and the baby's head, perfectly round because she hasn't done battle with the birth canal, will be lifted out first and her mouth and nose suctioned. As your doctor helps your baby out of the incision, you'll feel a strange pulling sensation. Once the cord is cut you'll be able to finally see your baby, although perhaps briefly, before she is taken for assessment and a quick cleanup by the nursing staff. Your incision will be stitched closed, and you'll be wheeled off to the recovery room where your little one will meet up with you once again. The entire surgical procedure will only take about 30 to 45 minutes.

Emergency C-Section

If your C-section is performed under emergency circumstances, things could move quickly and you'll have fewer options. You may also be given a general anesthetic that will make you unconscious. Most dads are asked to step outside when general anesthesia has been administered, but you might want to talk to your doctor about special circumstances during childbirth.

Induction

In cases where you are definitely 41 weeks or further along and it seems as if your child has decided she is perfectly content with spending her infancy in your womb, your practitioner may recommend induction. Inducing labor involves both helping the cervix ripen for baby's passage and stimulating uterine contractions. Both are important for a successful labor and delivery; if the cervix is not adequately effaced and dilated the chance of interventions (e.g., C-section or use of forceps) increases.

Your provider may use one of several methods to facilitate cervical ripening, including membrane stripping and amniotomy (manual breaking of the membranes or "bag of waters"). Stripping, or sweeping, of the membranes is simply the separation of the amniotic membrane from the wall of the cervix. Your provider will insert her finger in the cervix and gently sweep it between the amniotic membrane and the uterine wall.

If she opts for amniotomy, she'll use an instrument with a small blunt hook on the end (an amnihook) to break through the amniotic sac. With the latter method, if labor does not start on its own within 24 hours, scheduled induction may be necessary because of the risk of infection for the baby.

Because a scheduled induction is more successful when the cervix is prepared for the experience, your practitioner may recommend an application of prostaglandin gel to your cervix the day prior. The prostaglandin helps to ripen the cervix for labor and delivery. In some cases, it may be used alone as an inducing agent. The gel is applied to your vagina with a swab while the baby's heart rate is assessed with a fetal monitor. More than one application may be ordered.

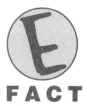

FACT

A study published in the journal *Obstetrics & Gynecology* in 2002 found that the rate of labor induction in the United States more than doubled between 1989 and 1998. And according to the U.S. Centers for Disease Control (CDC) more than one in five births were induced in 2001. Researchers attribute the increase to earlier prenatal care, wider availability of induction agents, and non-medical reasons such as convenience for the patient or doctor. Because induction can cause intense contractions and result in a longer labor, its use should always be carefully considered.

Pitocin—a synthetic formulation of the hormone oxytocin that stimulates uterine contractions—may be prescribed as an inducing agent. The hormone is given intravenously, and you will be hooked up to a fetal monitor to monitor your baby's progress.

After Birth

The pinnacle of 9 months of physical chaos and emotional oscillation, of queasy stomachs, lost car keys, aches, pains, and hair-trigger laughter and tears, has arrived. Your baby is here, placed skin to skin to feel her mother's outside warmth for the very first time.

Meeting Baby

A thousand different feelings and emotions, from utter exhaustion to indescribable joy, will flood you as you look down at that little scrunched face, still adjusting to its new waterless environment. Wrapped in a blanket with a little stocking cap to keep her head warm, she looks so perfect yet so vulnerable.

If you're planning on breastfeeding, you can nurse her while you get acquainted, or even in the recovery room if you've had a C-section. It's awe-inspiring how she knows just what to do, instinctively rooting for your breast with her eyes barely open, and then latching on. Spend as long as you want getting familiar and let baby's daddy share in the bonding, too. This is a precious time for your new family.

Baby's First "Doctor's Visit"

After you've met your child, he'll need some initial tests and treatments to ensure a healthy welcome into the world. The first is an Apgar test, which is simply an assessment of baby's reactivity, health, and appearance at birth. Created by noted pediatrician Dr. Virginia Apgar, the Apgar measures Appearance (skin color), Pulse, Grimace (reflexes), Activity, and Respiration. The Apgar is given just 1 minute after birth, and again 5 minutes after that. The attendant will assign a score of 0 to 2 for each category and add them together for the total Apgar. An average score is 7 to 10.

After the Apgar, your newborn will be measured, weighed, and have prints taken of his feet and fingers. Silver nitrate or antibiotic eyedrops or ointment may be put in his eyes to prevent infection from anything he encountered in the birth canal. He'll also receive a vitamin K injection to prevent bleeding problems; a heelstick blood draw to test for PKU and hypothyroidism; and in some hospitals a hepatitis B vaccine. Further tests may be administered if you have a chronic illness or experienced complications during pregnancy. If you have diabetes, for example, your newborn will have his blood glucose (sugar) levels tested.

Taking Care of Mom

After the birth, you'll have some assistance cleaning up and will be given a good supply of super absorbent sanitary pads. You'll also be provided with a peribottle, a plastic squirt bottle used to cleanse and soothe your perineal area with warm water each time you use the bathroom.

You'll be expelling lochia for up to 6 weeks following birth, whether you've had a vaginal birth or a C-section. Lochia—a mixture of blood, mucus, and tissue that comes from the site of implantation of the placenta—will be quite heavy in the days immediately following the birth, so don't be alarmed.

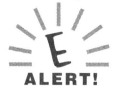

ALERT!

If bleeding is soaking through more than a pad per hour let your provider know. It could be a sign that a piece of placenta is still retained in your uterus.

If you've had a C-section, you'll spend some time in the recovery area before heading to your hospital room. Your incision will be checked regularly and pain medication will be administered as needed. The next day, you'll be encouraged to walk as soon as possible to get your digestive tract active again, and you'll be asked about your gas and bathroom habits ad nauseum. The nursing staff is just trying to ensure everything is returning to normal in gastrointestinal land.

Women who are given episiotomies will take sitz baths (also known as hip baths) to relieve pain, promote healing, and keep the area clean. A sitz bath is a small shallow tub of water, sometimes with medication added, that you sit in. Some mild pain relievers may also be prescribed to ease episiotomy pain.

Hospital Stay

Many hospitals have rooming in, where your baby can sleep in your hospital room with you and you can begin the process of learning to care and comfort him. It's a marvelous way to promote early bonding. However, if you are exhausted and your little guy seems to be having a problem getting to sleep, don't hesitate to get some help from the nursing staff. If you need a nap, they can wheel him down to the nursery for a few hours while you sleep. Childbirth, whether vaginally or by C-section, takes a physical toll that you need to recover from in order to parent effectively.

For the same reason, don't feel bad about keeping visitors to a minimum. Your hospital will have a visitor's policy, which will help somewhat. While introducing immediate family to their new relative is important, friends, neighbors, and coworkers can wait. At many facilities, you can also request that the switchboard hold phone calls to your room. Anyone who has a cold or other infection, even a family member, should not come in contact with your baby right now because of the risk of infection, and hand washing is a must for all visitors. Her little immune system is just starting to rev up.

For more on introducing siblings to their new brother or sister, see Chapter 11.

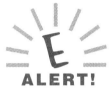

ALERT!

Recovery from a C-section will take a bit longer than from a vaginal delivery. When you laugh, sneeze, or cough, hold onto your incision with both hands. You'll find that using extra pillows for support over the incision area will allow you to cuddle and breastfeed your baby in comfort.

If you are planning on breastfeeding, now is the perfect time to get your technique down. Your OB nurses will likely ask you how breastfeeding is progressing, and they may request that you write down the time and frequency of nursing so they can assess baby's progress. They can also examine your latching technique to help you troubleshoot if things aren't yet going smoothly. In some cases, there may even be a lactation consultant available, and hospitals frequently offer breastfeeding classes to their new mother inpatients. For more on breastfeeding, see Chapter 19.

Remember that while it will take a few days for your breasts to start manufacturing milk, you are still providing your child with nutrient-rich colostrum, the prelude to breast milk. When your milk does arrive (or "come in"), about the third day after delivery, your breasts may be quite swollen, hard, and sore. This engorgement will be relieved upon nursing. If you're going the bottle route, cold packs and supportive bras or binding can ease the discomfort. The tenderness of engorgement usually passes in 2 to 3 days and may be relieved by mild analgesics as prescribed by your doctor. While you wait for your milk supply to dry up again (usually a period of about 2 weeks), you can use nursing pads to prevent leaks.

On Your Mind

Mortified by the possibility of losing control—both physically and emotionally—during labor? Childbirth is hard, painful work, and you need to work through it in your own way. The people around you are medical professionals and know this. Pain, and the ultimate goal of meeting your child, is a great motivator for getting past feelings of fear or bashfulness.

Many women who were once shy or self-conscious about their body find that pregnancy and motherhood pretty much eradicate any lingering traces of modesty they may have once had. When you're in labor you don't care if the attending doctor is animal, vegetable, or mineral; your mind and body are entirely focused on the impending arrival of your child. After they've been through the birth experience, many women find that there's virtually nothing that can embarrass them.

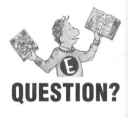

QUESTION?

Should we have our son circumcised?
The American Association of Pediatrics takes the stance that there is currently no firm medical or hygienic grounds for performing routine circumcision in newborn boys. However, the AAP also cited the importance of weighing cultural and religious beliefs and the child's best interest into the decision to circumcise or not. If circumcision is performed, analgesia should be used to relieve the pain. The AAP recommends a lidocaine nerve block as the most effective method currently available, but you should talk to your pediatrician about options.

Just for Dads

Until today, your most important function may have seemed to be back rubs and the Saturday night cheesecake run. But as labor starts, you will see just how pivotal your presence is in the childbirth process.

Coaching Your Team

You'll wear a number of hats as coach—gopher, massage therapist, hall monitor, motivational speaker, and advocate. Your partner must focus completely on the task at hand, and she will rely on your support for quashing distractions and attending to her needs.

Don't be offended if you're told to take your stopwatch and cram it, or if she impatiently shoos you away as you try to regulate her breathing. She still wants you, and more importantly needs you, by her side. Be flexible, stick with it, and work with her toward your common goal of a beautiful healthy baby.

Reassurance for the Faint of Heart

Birth, both by C-section and vaginally, can be a very blood-soaked scene. Chances are the rush of seeing your baby emerge will overwhelm any aversions to blood and other bodily fluids. But if it doesn't, don't feel bad about taking a moment to collect yourself—outside the room if need be. A nurse or another support person can stand in for you in the meantime. Now is not the time to faint, fall, and get a concussion (although many an expectant dad has passed out in the heat of the moment). One tip—if you are known for getting the whim-whams at the sight of blood, you and your partner should discuss the possibility of your early exit before labor. You may want to have a stand-by coach just in case.

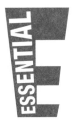

If your partner is having a C-section, there will be a surgical curtain or drape positioned above her belly. Typically dad is positioned by mom's head for emotional support throughout the procedure. To avoid the sight of blood, and your significant other's internal organs, simply stay below the sight line of the surgical drape by remaining seated on a stool by your partner's head. If the attending nurse hasn't given you a seat, request one.

The Best Laid Plans

Things can go wrong in childbirth, but the more you know about complications in advance, the easier it is to deal with them should they arise.

Emergency Birth

In cases where the fetus begins to show signs of distress (rapid acceleration or sudden slowdown of fetal heart rate) or you experience a life-threatening condition such as hemorrhage, you will be rushed to the OR for an emergency caesarean. In most cases, because time is of the essence, you will be given a general anesthetic.

Women who attempt a vaginal birth after caesarean (VBAC) may be at risk for uterine rupture or a separation of their previous C-section scar. If this occurs, an emergency C-section would be performed. It should be noted, however, that the success rate of VBAC is very good—between 60 and 80 percent of individuals who are considered candidates for the procedure come through it with flying colors.

Delivery Complications

A child with a head too large for passage through the pelvis (called cephalopelvic disproportion), a labor that fails to progress past 6 or 7 centimeters despite all best efforts, or fetal distress caused by a compressed umbilical cord are all possible complications that could cause an unplanned caesarean section.

In some cases, where your baby may need a little extra help getting out of the birth canal, the use of forceps may be required. This tong-like device is used to reach into the birth canal, gently grasp the baby's head, and pull him out. Forceps are also used to reposition a baby who is intent on arriving in a poor position.

Sometimes forceps are simply used to lift the baby up and out right there at your perineum, which is called perineal use or outlet forceps. Babies delivered via forceps do wear signs of these instruments as bruises or red marks on either side of their heads for a few days and there is a very slim risk of brain injury.

If your provider is concerned that using forceps will injure your perineal tissues, he may choose vacuum extraction instead. Suctioned onto the baby's head, the cup is attached to a chain that the doctor pulls on while you keep on pushing. The cup will simply fall off the baby's head if too much pressure builds up. However, babies who arrive via vacuum extraction can have a bruised, swollen look to the top of their heads.

Other maternal complications may occur following a successful delivery. Postpartum hemorrhage and a related dive in blood pressure can occur when the uterus fails to contract again after both baby and placenta have been delivered. Compression and massage of the uterus and/or drug therapy may be used to stop the bleeding. In cases where a tear of the cervix has occurred, it will be sutured. If these measures still don't stop the bleeding, surgery may be required.

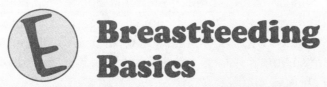

Chapter 19

Breastfeeding Basics

Breastfeeding is one part instinct, one part practice, and a whole lot of persistence and patience. It's that last part that makes the difference between breast and bottle for many women, particularly in the first weeks of motherhood when even minor nursing difficulties may seem insurmountable. The good news is that breastfeeding usually becomes easier and more fulfilling over time.

Breast or Bottle?

Are you going to breastfeed or go the formula route? It's an issue that many new moms feel intensely pressured about, and if you're still undecided you've likely heard extensive opinions on the subject. Which is the right choice?

If you were comparing breast milk to formula strictly on a nutrient basis, few would disagree that the best choice is breast milk. But since the issue is also loaded with social, emotional, and personal considerations, things are seldom so black and white. In the end, breast or bottle is an individual choice.

Pros and Cons

One woman's plus is another's "no way." Consider the pros and cons to breast and bottle feeding, and how they fit into your particular life and family situation.

Breastfeeding pros and cons

PRO: The hands-down perfect food for your child, breast milk is custom made specifically for her nutritional needs and provides her with essential antibodies.
CON: If you have a medical condition that requires drug treatment, it's possible your medication may pass into breast milk and potentially pose a risk to baby (talk with your doctor if this is the case; you may have other treatment options).

PRO: Breastfeeding is a low-maintenance feeding routine. It's always close at hand and never needs mixing, warming, or other preparation.
CON: In the beginning, at least, you will always need to be close at hand as well. Breastfeeding can be as physically taxing as it is emotionally rewarding.

PRO: Nursing gives you special one-on-one bonding time with baby.
CON: Breasts don't detach. No one else can pitch in on the feeding duties.

PRO: If you're on a budget, breastfeeding is a big cost-cutter. Aside from the high cost of formula itself, you can save on bottles, bags, cleaning gadgets, and other formula feeding purchases.

CON: You may have to purchase or rent a breast pump and buy a personal kit to use with it, which can also be costly.

PRO: As a breastfeeding mom, you're taking part in a tradition as old as motherhood itself and giving your child something no one else can. The experience is priceless.

CON: Unfortunately, there are still many unenlightened knuckleheads out there that can't get past their perception of the breast as strictly a sexual object and who will relegate you to the corner or better yet, the closet, if given the chance.

PRO: Many women who breastfeed experience faster postpartum weight loss.

CON: Although you may be taking your figure back, your breasts belong to baby, leaks, sore nipples, and all.

Bottle feeding pros and cons

PRO: Feeding isn't only mom, all day and all night. Your partner can get up at 4 A.M. once in a while to feed the baby.

CON: Feeding isn't only mom, all day and all night. The special mother-child bond and skin-to-skin contact that breastfeeding brings may be harder to achieve.

PRO: You can give your baby a bottle just about anywhere, anytime without feeling self-conscious or raising eyebrows.

CON: Before you hit the road, make sure you've packed sterilized bottles and nipples, formula, bottled water for mixing powdered formula, a can opener for opening premixed formula, and an ice pack if you've made the bottles in advance. If they are chilled, you need a place to warm them, and don't forget the extra formula in case you're gone longer than you anticipated. Convenience is in the eye of the beholder.

PRO: No worries about keeping up your milk supply when you return to work.

CON: You may miss out on a golden opportunity to spend special nursing time together at home once your busy work schedule starts encroaching on family time again.

PRO: You can assume control of your body again, after many months away from the helm.

CON: After so many months as one, you're suddenly severing a close physical bond that nursing can prolong.

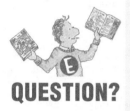

QUESTION?

I can't nurse when I return to work in 6 weeks. Should I even bother breastfeeding, or will my baby get confused?
Even a short period of breastfeeding can have big advantages for your baby, so whatever time you can commit he will benefit from. However, completely and abruptly weaning him from the breast cold turkey at 6 weeks will be tough on both of you. Keep in mind that many women return to work and continue to nurse, either by pumping or simply reducing the number of feedings from the breast so nursing is in the morning and the evening, and the baby is supplemented with formula at other times.

Being Comfortable with Your Decision

You are not an uncaring and self-absorbed mother if you choose to bottle-feed. Likewise, if you breastfeed your child openly and even through toddlerhood you are not a mother-earth militant nut.

Try to weigh the risks versus the benefits in your situation. All other things being equal, women who are well-supported at home, are healthy, and don't face an excessively demanding work schedule should consider giving breastfeeding a try even if they feel a little awkward about it. Often the awkwardness evaporates with a little practice and the bond forged with baby in nursing. And the health benefits gained by baby will last a lifetime.

On the other hand, if you're a single mom who works two jobs and is already stretched to the limit emotionally and physically, don't be pressured into breastfeeding by others because it is "the right thing to do." Excessive stress can do more damage than good, impairing your parenting skills, putting your health at risk, and straining the time the two of you do have together. Not every life situation is ideal for breastfeeding, even if you are capable of doing it. Make the decision that works best for your family.

Your Body and Breastfeeding

As soon as you can hold baby, you can breastfeed her. In the first few days following birth, your breasts will produce a clear to yellow sticky substance called colostrum. Colostrum contains antibodies that help strengthen the infant immune system. It also is important for getting baby's digestion off on the right track. The low-carbohydrate, high-protein concoction is easily digestible for these early days and helps to establish intestinal flora, a beneficial bacteria, in baby's gastrointestinal tract. It also encourages the passing of meconium, your infant's first stools.

Colostrum comes out in small amounts compared to later breast milk, which will fill the alvoeli, or milk ducts, of your breast about 3 days after birth. You'll know when your milk "comes in"—your breasts will become engorged with milk, rock hard, and sore to the touch. Nursing your baby will relieve the pressure quickly, although it's possible you may need a little additional help to ease soreness. A few clinical studies have shown some benefit in the use of cabbage leaves (yes, cabbage leaves) to relieve the discomfort of engorgement. Massage and warm compresses can also help.

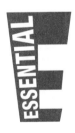

Sore or dry and cracked nipples are a common phenomenon as you get off the breastfeeding launch pad. Never fear—they will "toughen up." In the meantime, try vitamin E oil for moisturizing, or lanolin ointment for easing abrasions and pain. With the lanolin, a little goes a long, long way. You'll only need a tiny dollop with each, and one tube will probably last you through infancy, toddlerhood, and possibly beyond.

Latching and Letdown

Some babies seem to be breastfeeding champs from the get-go, and others need a little coaching. You're both new at this, so have patience and remember that you'll get better with practice. If you're having a hospital stay after your birth, the nurses on the maternity ward can give you some pointers on technique and check baby's latch. In some cases, there may even be a lactation specialist on staff to consult with.

Start with a comfortable position for the two of you. Baby's whole body should face yours, not just her turned head. The cradle and cross-cradle holds are two common positions. The cradle holds your baby close across the front of your body, with her head in the crook of your arm and your hand supporting her bottom. The cross-cradle switches arms and puts your hand under her head. Lying down with baby facing you is a good choice for the utterly exhausted.

The football position (or clutch hold) tucks baby under your arm, again facing your body and breast. If you've had a C-section, this can help by keeping the weight off your incision. It's also a favorite of moms with twins for doing double nursing duty (see Chapter 7 for tips on breast-feeding multiples). The seated Australian hold might be a good choice if you'd like to try to keep baby awake during and after his feeding. With all nursing positions, make sure your baby's head is well supported.

After you're settled into position, brace your breast with one hand, cupped into the shape of a "C." If you have small breasts, this may not be necessary after a time, but try the C-hold initially to make sure baby latches on correctly.

Encouraging baby to get a successful latch is the most important part of the process. Stroke her bottom lip with your nipple until she opens her mouth wide and yawn-like. This is called the rooting reflex. Insert your nipple into her mouth and she should instinctively close, or latch, onto it.

A proper latch:

- Encompasses the entire nipple and most, if not all, of the areola.
- Positions her nose almost directly on your breast (she can breathe, don't worry).
- Can be verified by her visible and possibly audible swallowing.
- Will *not* hurt (unless the nipple is in poor condition to begin with).

Cradle hold

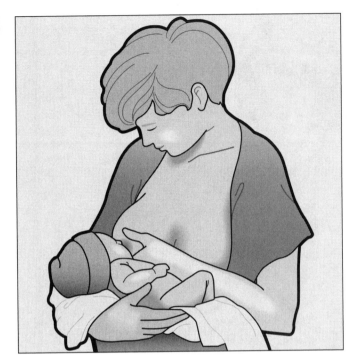

◀ Choose a comfortable nursing position that works for both of you, and make sure baby's head is well supported.

Cross-cradle hold

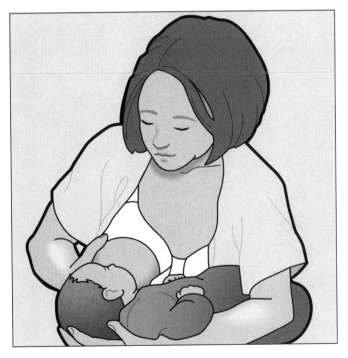

Football clutch hold

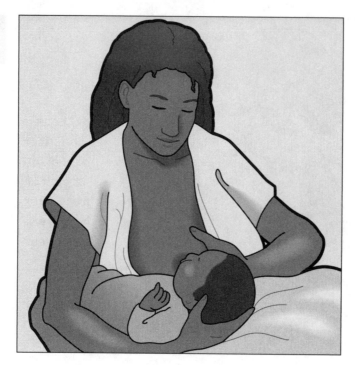

Side lying hold

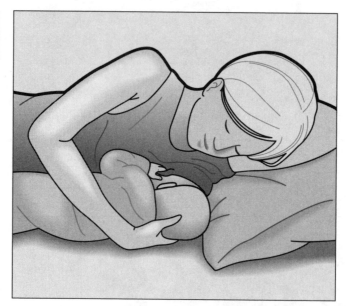

Australian hold

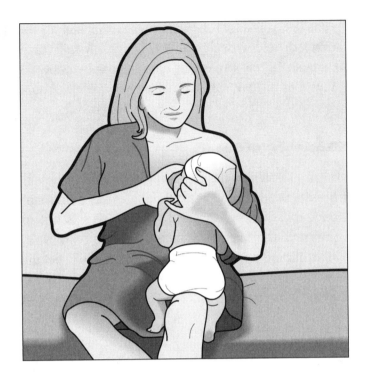

C-hold

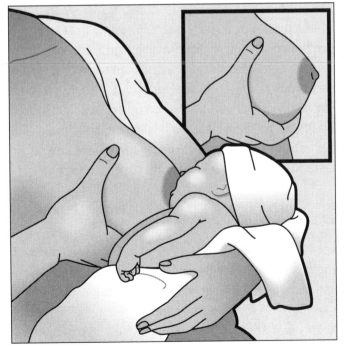

◀ Use the C-hold to support your breast for baby and encourage a proper latch.

As your baby nurses, you'll feel a warm tingling that signals the milk ejection reflex (MER), or letdown. The feeling is actually milk being released into the sinuses of the breast for easy access by baby. Some women don't always feel the MER, but you'll know when it occurs if your baby suddenly picks up his pace of sucking and swallowing.

Supply and Demand System

When everything operates as designed, the more baby nurses, the more milk your breasts produce. A breast that baby has completely drained will produce milk at a faster rate than one that has only been partially empty. Your milk production takes its cue from baby. So if your child is premature or ill and isn't nursing, or is latching or sucking ineffectively, your milk supply will adjust downward. A breast pump can help keep the milk flowing until baby is ready to nurse full time again.

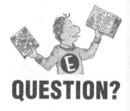

QUESTION?

Will this kid ever stop eating? It seems like I'm nursing constantly!
Newborns don't believe much in schedules, do they? In some cases, constant nursing in a fussy baby might indicate an insufficient milk supply. But as long as he's growing fine and is having six to eight wet diapers and about three dirty diapers daily, you can be assured he's getting plenty to eat. Nursing 10 to 12 times a day is also normal for a newborn. Just bear with it and as the weeks pass and he develops, he'll spend more time exploring and less time eating. In the meantime, his frequent snacks are helping to establish and grow your milk supply, which is great.

Practical Matters

Button-up blouses, shirts with zippers, and other easy-access clothing will make nursing easier on a day-to-day basis. There are a variety of different nursing bras available; make sure you try them on before purchase to ensure a good fit. You may opt for the comfort of a simple jogging or sports bra that slides up easily, especially if you like the added support of wearing a bra to bed.

Nursing pads for catching leaks before they soak through your shirt are also a must. These come in several different materials and configurations, including cloth, plastic, and disposable. Disposable has the advantage of high absorbency, while cloth can be washed and reused. Accidents do happen, even with pads, and carrying an extra shirt in your bag or car may save you a mortifying moment or two.

Every nursing mother could use a good breastfeeding reference book for guidance. *The Womanly Art of Breastfeeding* from La Leche League International is considered the breastfeeding bible by many. *The New Mothers' Guide to Breastfeeding* from the American Academy of Pediatrics is also a useful resource.

Baby's Body and Breastfeeding

Trying to impose a strict feeding schedule on your newborn will result in much heartache and little success. Unless you have multiples, there's really no good reason to start scheduling baby's meals at specific times. If you do have twins or more, you may want to wake them all when one gets up for a feeding to get them on a similar routine, but that still doesn't mean feeding by the clock. Only your baby can determine how much he needs to satisfy his tummy, and feeding on demand is the best way to accomplish this.

The health rewards for your nursing child's body and mind are tremendous. Breast milk improves immunity, is thought to offer protection against certain chronic diseases (e.g., type 1 diabetes), is associated with a reduced risk of SIDS, and is easy on baby's digestive system. Clinical studies have also indicated that breastfeeding may boost baby's brainpower and can enhance cognitive development in small for gestational age (SGA) babies.

So how long do you breastfeed for? From a clinical standpoint, the American Academy of Pediatrics (AAP) has recommended breastfeeding for at least one year and as long as both mother and child are still comfortable with the arrangement thereafter. The best answer is probably as long as both of you are still enjoying and benefiting from it.

Bottle Basics

If you do choose to bottle feed, there are literally hundreds of bottle types and nipple configurations on the market. Figuring out what works and what doesn't is largely trial and error, but there are some things you can look for:

- **Low air flow.** Designs that minimize air or can be de-aired prior to feeding may reduce baby's gas.
- **Convenience.** If saving time is a priority, features like presterilized disposable bag bottles are a big plus.
- **Easy to clean.** Pick something with minimal parts that looks easy to clean and sterilize.
- **Built for baby.** Get a newborn-style nipple with a smaller opening to start so baby doesn't face a formula tidal wave. If her sucking reflex is weak, you may have to upgrade to a larger opening.

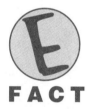

FACT

Baby's digestive system is still immature, and his tiny stomach can only hold 2 to 4 teaspoons of fluid at birth. For this reason, you'll notice spit-up is a frequent event. Don't be alarmed. It's his signal that the tank is full. Swallowing air and too much activity with a full tummy can also cause spitting up. However, if baby's spit-up becomes excessive and forceful (projectile vomiting), or is accompanied by gagging or difficulty swallowing, call your pediatrician immediately. It could be a sign that your baby has a formula intolerance or a gastrointestinal problem.

For women who are breastfeeding and need to introduce a bottle, look for a nipple variety that mimics the natural contours of the breast. Your baby may be less likely to balk at a bottle that feels similar to you.

Both breastfed and bottle-fed babies require regular burping during a meal. You'll quickly pick up your child's cues that a bubble needs bursting; she may arch her back and fuss at the breast or bottle. In the beginning, burping at least twice during a feeding session can help to ensure her comfort.

Seated

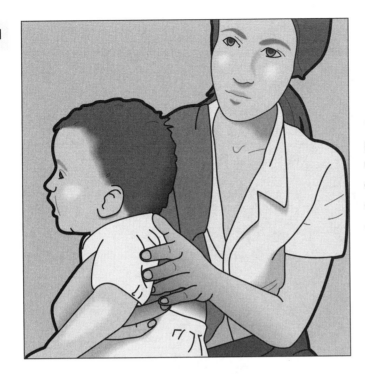

◀ There are several positions you can use to burp baby effectively: seated, over the shoulder, and across the lap.

Seated

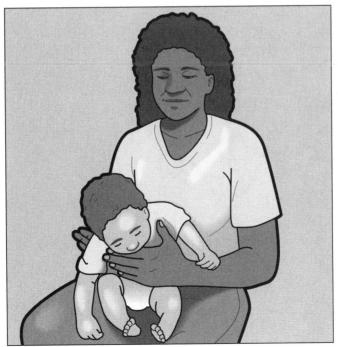

Over the
shoulder

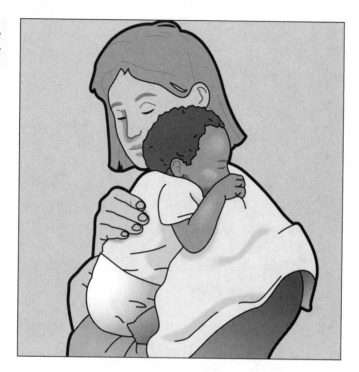

Across the lap

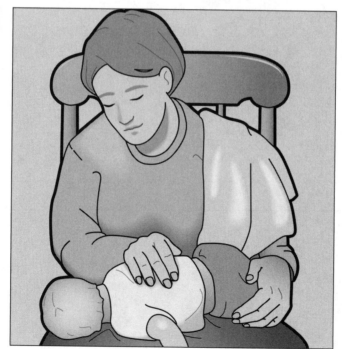

Eating Right: For Mom

A pattern of healthy eating in pregnancy will continue to reward you and baby now that you're breastfeeding. Keep up the same routine with healthy food choices and plenty of noncaffeinated fluids (8 to 12 glasses a day).

Nursing burns approximately 500 calories per day, but that doesn't mean you will need to bulk up your diet significantly. Your body has plenty to spare and has stored extra fat for the very purpose of lactation. The American Dietetic Association recommends following the modified breastfeeding food pyramid.

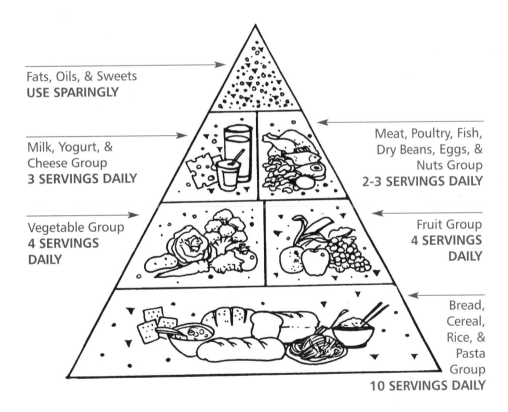

Fats, Oils, & Sweets
USE SPARINGLY

Milk, Yogurt, &
Cheese Group
3 SERVINGS DAILY

Meat, Poultry, Fish,
Dry Beans, Eggs, &
Nuts Group
2-3 SERVINGS DAILY

Vegetable Group
**4 SERVINGS
DAILY**

Fruit Group
**4 SERVINGS
DAILY**

Bread,
Cereal,
Rice, &
Pasta
Group
10 SERVINGS DAILY

▲ The modified USDA food pyramid for breastfeeding mothers adds an extra serving from each food group.

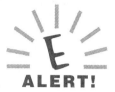

ALERT!

Even though you may be tempted to cut calories drastically in order to get your old body back, now is not the time to crash diet. Losing weight too quickly can release excessive levels of any toxins like pesticides and PCBs that reside in your maternal fat stores, which will consequently pass into breast milk. Also stay away from extremely low carbohydrate diets right now, as they can cause ketosis, another potential danger to a nursing baby.

On Your Mind

Breastfeeding doesn't come naturally to everyone. Ingrained feelings of self-consciousness about your body, of modesty, and of discomfort with the process may inhibit your natural inclination to nurse. When things don't go according to plan and the nursing relationship isn't thriving, feelings of inadequacy are common. Seeking assistance, either through coaching or supplemental nutrition, is not a sign of failure but rather of dedication to your child. Breastfeeding, in any amount, is something to take tremendous pride in.

Breasts: From Form to Function

Where is the right spot to nurse? Wherever your baby is hungry. As long as it's done as discreetly as circumstances warrant, there shouldn't be any place that's appropriate to bring a baby to that isn't also an appropriate place to breastfeed.

The thought of nursing in public may be worrying you. When the time comes, don't think about your exposure, think only of filling your child's stomach. A baby who's really singing for his supper will probably not give you the time to be modest about it anyway.

Specially designed nursing blankets can improve your cover if you're really self-conscious, although a receiving blanket over the shoulder works as well. If you do use one of these, make sure they're comfortable and not too hot for baby.

Support from Family and Friends

Breastfeeding doesn't always come naturally and immediately, particularly for first-time moms. Having the support of your friends and family is really important in making it through those first few uncertain and sometimes rocky weeks. Comments like, "Why don't you just give her a bottle?" will do nothing but erode your confidence and stress you out. Get your partner's help in deflecting the negativity and explaining your reasons for breastfeeding, but if the bad attitudes continue, just avoid the offender. You don't need it.

A La Leche League group can also be a steadfast source of support and inspiration, and more importantly, guidance for your breastfeeding difficulties. Call ✆ 1-800-LALECHE for a group in your area or see Appendix A for further contact information.

Lactation Problems

Learning to read baby's body language and vocal cues is an acquired art, one that takes time to acclimate to. It's easy to miss hunger signals, or mistake them for other needs. For now, familiarize yourself with the warning signs of insufficient feeding. If your baby is having fewer than six wet and three dirty diapers a day, is excessively fussy at the breast, has a sunken fontanel (soft spot), acts lethargic, and is not at or above birth weight by 2 weeks postpartum (or steadily gaining thereafter), he is probably not getting enough, and needs to see his pediatrician immediately. Fortunately, with some work and a little guidance, you should both be able to get back on track.

Why Your Body Isn't Cooperating

There are dozens of reasons why milk supply or nursing itself may not be making the cut, but most of them can be overcome with patience, special equipment, and/or professional training and guidance.

- **Medication:** Antihistamines, decongestants, contraceptives, and some other medications can have a detrimental effect on milk supply. Talk to your doctor before taking any medication while nursing.

- **Inverted nipples:** If you have inverted nipples, a good latch may be elusive. Breast shields designed to pull the nipple out can help.
- **Prior breast surgery:** Many women nurse successfully after breast surgery, but certain types of breast augmentation (enlargement) or breast reduction surgery do have the potential to hinder your milk supply depending on how they are performed. Talk to your doctor if you've had breast surgery and are having lactation problems.
- **Hypotrophic breast disease:** Some women have structural problems with the breast tissue that decreases the number of milk-producing ducts. You may still be able to nurse, but baby may require supplemental feedings. Again, speak with your provider about your options.
- **Retained placental fragment:** Lactation problems can be a sign that a piece of your placenta was missed in delivery. Since this can also cause severe hemorrhage, suspected retained placenta should be assessed by your provider immediately.
- **Stress:** New motherhood and all its related stressors can inhibit milk supply, and tension can make letdown (milk ejection) difficult. If you're uptight about nursing problems, the cycle perpetuates itself. Try to look forward to nursing as a relaxing, *de*-stressing time.
- **Poor technique:** Letting baby empty one breast before moving on to the next will stimulate milk supply and allow her to reach the fatty and filling hindmilk that is at the end of her "drink."
- **Poor nutrition and hydration:** Good eating habits and plenty of water are essential to your milk production efforts.
- **Nipple confusion:** The mechanics of drinking from a bottle are very different from those of feeding from the breast. If a bottle is introduced before breastfeeding is well established, it's possible for your baby to develop a preference for it.

Babies born prematurely, those with a poor sucking reflex, or those with a cleft lip or other health problem can have problems nursing initially. If your baby needs supplemental feeding in the hospital for any reason, you can request that it be administered with an eyedropper, syringe, feeding cup, or supplemental feeding system to avoid nipple confusion. You should also talk with your pediatrician and a lactation consultant about adaptive techniques and other options.

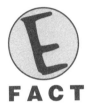

FACT

Breastfeeding problems with your first baby may have you wary to try it again. Keep in mind that just like every pregnancy and baby is different, nursing success can be too. Environmental factors play a large role in breastfeeding, so if the stress of your firstborn, coupled with the unprecedented exhaustion of that period, had your body in a tailspin, there's a good chance this time may be different. You also have the added benefit of experience on your side this time around. Don't be afraid to try again—if it doesn't work out, you still have options.

Lactation Consultants

A lactation consultant is a health care provider who specializes in breastfeeding support and training. If you're having difficulties with nursing, a consultant can be a huge help in helping you overcome breastfeeding difficulties. Your ob-gyn or your child's pediatrician can provide a referral if needed. Some large pediatric practices retain lactation consultants on staff.

A board certified lacation consultant will have the designation IBCLC (International Board Certified Lactation Consultant), which means he or she meets specific eligibility and experience requirements and has passed a board examination administered by the International Board of Lactation Consultant Examiners (IBLCE). Sometimes consultants are nurses who have earned board certification.

Many certified lactation consultants are also La Leche League leaders. Don't overlook the value of La Leche League support if you don't have a lactation consultant in your area. The organization can be a tremendous source of emotional support as well as practical advice and experience.

Pump Primer

A breast pump can be useful in ramping up your milk production if you're having supply issues. It's also a great tool for moms heading back to work who want to keep nursing, and for mothers of babies who are temporarily unable to nurse because of various health issues.

A pump may be manual (hand-powered) or a battery or electric unit. The hand-powered pumps have the advantage of being inexpensive and portable, but may take some getting used to and take longer to empty a breast. They use a piston-like action or a squeeze bulb to create the suction that removes the milk from your breast.

Hospital-grade electric units are probably the most efficient and allow you to pump both breasts at the same time, but are bulky to transport and costly to purchase. Weekly or monthly rental units are frequently available through lactation consultants, hospital programs, or private businesses. For safety reasons, you will have to purchase a personal kit for use with the rental unit that contains all the elements that come in contact with your breast milk, including tubing and bottles. The kit can be used for as long as you plan to pump, and usually runs around $20 to $30 for the basics.

Supplementing and Finger Feeding

If you're having breastfeeding problems, a supplemental nursing system (SNS) can help you provide baby with added nutrients of pumped breast milk or formula while still getting the benefits of suckling. A bottle or bag milk reservoir hangs around your neck, and two narrow silicone tubes channel milk flow from the reservoir to your nipple, where the open end of the tube is taped. As baby feeds on both the supplemental milk and breast milk you're providing, her suckling action also further stimulates your milk production.

Women who are having problems producing enough milk for whatever reason may be able to supplement from a local breast milk bank if one is nearby. Milk donors are screened for health problems in a process similar to blood donation screening. Again, a lactation consultant or pediatrician should have further information on what's available in your area.

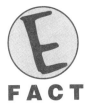

FACT

Finger feeding is similar in principle to an SNS, and is sometimes used as an alternative to an SNS. It uses a narrow feeding tube attached to a syringe or reservoir, in which breast milk or formula is placed. The other end of the tube is taped to your index or middle finger, and the baby gets her nourishment by sucking on your finger. If baby is not latching onto the breast for whatever reason (e.g., nipple confusion, separation from mom), finger feeding can provide nutrition without introducing a rubber nipple to the feeding process.

Mastitis

Mastitis is an infection of the breast that can be caused by a plugged milk duct. If you develop mastitis, you can and should keep nursing. Your baby cannot get ill from nursing from you during this time, and the breastfeeding process will actually help the mastitis resolve itself faster by easing the pain and draining the milk ducts.

Signs of mastitis include:

- Breast is warm to touch
- Red, tender streaks on the breast
- Pain and swelling
- Fever present

If you develop mastitis, stay on your nursing schedule and try to get sufficient rest to help your body heal. A warm water bottle, warm wet compress, or soaking in a hot shower may help to ease the discomfort. If the mastitis doesn't start to clear up in a day or so, or begins to worsen, you may need an antibiotic. Your health care provider can advise you as to what medications will be safe for breastfeeding.

Just for Dads

Although it may look easy, breastfeeding can be hard work, particularly the first time out. Your support is vital to this venture. Let your partner know you value this unique gift she's bestowing on your child. Be a voice of support when things get tough, and do what you can to create a warm and welcome environment for your nursing twosome. If the whole process has you bewildered, don't be embarrassed about asking questions.

Getting Comfortable with Breastfeeding

Be honest. Somewhere way in the back of your mind, or perhaps unabashedly front and center, you were a little freaked out at the concept of your partner as food source. If you weren't, more power to you, but it's normal to need a little time to adjust. Learning more about how beneficial breastfeeding is for your new baby may help increase your comfort level.

When you're both up to sex again, try to respect your partner's feelings about touching in the feeding zone. Nipple soreness, leaking milk, and breast sensitivity may have her feeling better left alone. Or she may be willing and you may be hesitant given whose mouth was there last. Whatever the situation, it's important you both get your current viewpoint out into the open so no one's feelings are hurt. Your outlook may evolve over time, or you may both decide to focus on other sources of pleasure.

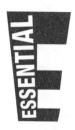

One thing you'll quickly learn about infant timing is that you'll be interrupted in the heat of passion at least once. When she returns from nursing baby, realize that switching gears from nurturing mommy to adventurous sex kitten can be a tall order to fill. Don't force the uncomfortable and awkward if the moment has passed for either of you. You won't have an infant forever, and this is just one of the many sudden detours of life that parenting brings.

Getting in on the Act

Just because your partner may be nursing doesn't cut you out of the feeding picture completely. At some point, after breastfeeding has been established, you will want to familiarize baby with a bottle of breast milk, in case mom's absence requires feeding her expressed milk.

Once a bottle is introduced, you can do the honors for a regular feeding. Some babies are hesitant to take a bottle from mom when they know her nice warm breast is just an arm's reach away, so your presence may be a necessity for this task.

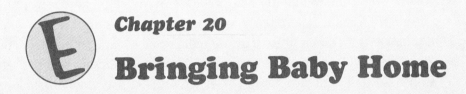

Chapter 20

Bringing Baby Home

The first days at home with your new family are fun but challenging. Your body is going through some intense physical changes. And if you thought those hormonal changes that pregnancy brought were now finished, well, think again. Enjoy this special time getting acquainted and settling into your new lifestyle.

Your Body Postpartum

From the moment your child slides out of your body, a transformation as dramatic as that of pregnancy begins. Right at delivery you will drop around 10 to 15 pounds of baby, placenta, amniotic fluid, and lochia.

By the tenth day postpartum, your incredible shrinking uterus will have contracted to one-twentieth of its prelabor size and the cervix will be closed once again. Afterpains similar to menstrual cramps and a steady discharge of lochia indicate that the uterus is returning to normal. The lochia flow will continue up to 6 weeks, but the afterpains will probably stop several days after delivery (although nursing may continue to stimulate them periodically).

Your perineal area may continue to be sore for a few weeks, particularly when you need to relieve yourself. Take your peribottle from the hospital home with you and keep it in the bathroom for regular use. A hot water bottle and occasional cold packs can also ease pain and swelling. If sitting is uncomfortable, you can purchase a foam "donut" for your chair at a medical supply store. Most stitches dissolve within a week and external ones may fall out. Pelvic floor exercises can help speed up the healing process.

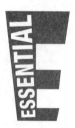

Lochia flow will be heavy and bright red at first, but the color will gradually change to pink and then yellow or brown. The flow will taper off within 10 to 14 days, although some discharge is normal for up to 6 weeks. However, the bright red color may begin again at times. If it does, take it as a sign that you may be doing too much too soon, and slow down. Never use tampons to control lochia flow because of the risk of infection.

As your body drops tissue, fluids, and decreases its cardiovascular volume, your metabolism may seem completely out of whack. Vaginally, things may seem a little "looser" in general. Your vaginal skin is quite elastic, and may be stretched out from the birth. Exercise and time will help it return to a firmer state.

Constipation is another common postpartum problem, primarily because of the loss of abdominal muscle tone and painkillers that can slow your digestive processes. Plenty of water, movement, and high-fiber foods may help. If you had a C-section, your incision may also make you hesitant to bear down very hard. Supporting it with a rolled up towel can help. A stool softener may be prescribed as well; check with your practitioner if you are breastfeeding before taking any medication.

Your breasts will be tender as you deal with engorgement. Women who aren't planning on nursing will find that drying up your milk supply fully can be a somewhat uncomfortable process. If you do breastfeed, sore nipples and other discomforts may be plaguing you as you adjust to this new routine.

Recovering after Caesarean

When you've had a C-section you're recovering from major surgery and need to treat yourself accordingly. Sleep when baby sleeps and stay away from strenuous activity and heavy lifting (nothing bigger than baby as a general rule). Use a bed pillow or a nursing pillow (Boppy) to hold your baby without pressuring your incision. Pain medication may be prescribed; if you're breastfeeding talk to your doctor about judicious use.

Your doctor will recommend 6 weeks of rest and recuperation (within limits—you are a new mom after all), and you'll be advised not to drive while taking pain medications. Second or subsequent C-section moms may recover a bit quicker, just because they know what to expect and treat themselves accordingly. Above all, don't push it, or you'll set your recovery back even further.

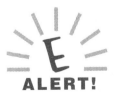

Women can and do get pregnant in the period following birth. Although sex may be the last thing on your mind at the moment, if you aren't up to a return to the delivery room in 9 or 10 short months, get back on a contraceptive routine now before the mood strikes. Your doctor can give you a prescription before you leave the hospital, if necessary. Abstain from intercourse for 4 to 6 weeks after delivery.

Baby's Body: An Operator's Manual

Your baby will actually lose weight as she starts out in life, but should be back up to birth weight by her 2-week checkup. Thereafter, she may put on 1 pound every 2 weeks, doubling her birth weight by month 4. Premature babies sometimes grow a little slower, but most will eventually catch up.

Her eyesight is a bit hazy, but she can see you fairly clearly when you hold her 7 to 10 inches away from your face. Studies show she knows your voice well already from listening to it in the womb, and prefers it to a stranger's.

Your newborn arrives with a variety of natural reflexes or involuntary ways of moving:

- **Palmar, or grasping, reflex.** When you touch your baby's open hand, she'll make a fist around your finger.
- **Rooting reflex.** If you stroke her cheek, her head will turn toward your touch. This reflex helps the bleary-eyed newborn find her food source, and you can use it to guide her to the breast or bottle.
- **Sucking reflex.** Once at the breast or bottle, baby's sucking reflex takes over as she automatically sucks on anything put in her mouth.
- **Startle, or moro, reflex.** When baby is startled, he will thrust his arms and legs out and arch his back, then quickly pull arms and legs in again.
- **Babinski reflex.** Stroking baby's foot will make him spread his toes and flex his foot in.
- **Stepping reflex.** Hold your baby up with your hands under her armpits so that her feet are touching a firm surface. She will lift her feet up and down like she is about to take baby steps.
- **Tonic neck reflex.** When placed on his back, baby turns his head to the right and makes fists with his hands.
- **Blinking.** The involuntary reflex of closing her eyes when they are exposed to bright light, air, or another stimulus is the one reflex that baby will keep for the rest of her life.

From Soft Spot to Curled Toes

The bones of baby's skull are not yet fused together, and unless you had a caesarean delivery your baby's head may look a bit, well, pointy. This cone-headed appearance is the result of pressure in the birth canal and will round out within a few weeks. There are four small areas on your baby's head where the baby's skull bones have not yet joined together, called fontanelles (or soft spots). Three of these fontanelles fuse within the first 4 months of life, but the longest lasting and most visible of these—the diamond-shaped area on the top of the head called the anterior fontanelle (or soft spot)—may take up to 18 months to close. Many a curious sibling has reached out to jab this pulsating spot, much to their parent's horror. Don't get too concerned—your baby's brain is well protected by a tough membrane called the dura mater.

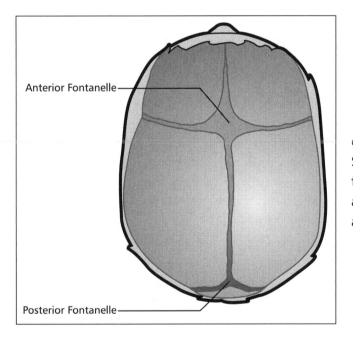

Anterior Fontanelle

Posterior Fontanelle

◀ Baby's soft spot is called a fontanelle. She has a total of four, but only the anterior and posterior are easily located.

The eye color your baby has at birth may change later in infancy or childhood. This is due to the ongoing production of the hormone melanin, which can cause later eye color changes.

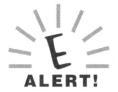

ALERT!

If the fontanelle ever appears deeply sunken or bulging, call your baby's pediatrician immediately. A sunken soft spot is a sign of dehydration, or your baby not getting sufficient fluids. And a fontanelle that bulges could be an indication of increased pressure in the brain from fluid buildup or hemorrhage. Keep in mind that crying can make the fontanelle appear swollen. A normal fontanelle is slightly curved in and soft yet firm to the touch.

Baby's Skin

Your newborn's soft-as-butter skin may have some imperfections at first. Post-term babies are more likely to have some peeling, while preterm babies may still be sporting a substantial amount of lanugo and vernix. Although the vernix is fairly well rubbed off by the time you bring baby home, you may continue to find it in his creases and crevices until his first real bath. The lanugo will rub itself off over the next few weeks.

Baby may also be wearing one or more birthmarks on his birthday suit. Red marks on the eyelids, forehead, and at the very back of the nape of the neck usually fade and disappear over time and are called salmon patches or stork bites. Red, strawberry birthmarks can increase in size but may shrink and be gone by age five. Your baby may also have one or more light brown birthmarks known as café au lait spots. Very rarely, café au lait spots (particularly a large number of marks) are symptomatic of one of several uncommon medical conditions. Talk to your child's doctor if you have any concerns.

Dark blue to blue-green spots on the buttocks or lower back are known as Mongolian spots. They are most common in African-American, Native American, and Asian newborns and fade over time. If your baby is born with what is known as a port wine stain, a bright red or purple mark that is considered to be more permanent, plastic surgery is an option in later life if they are located in a prominent spot. Ask your pediatrician or family doctor for more information.

Little whiteheads called milia are common on newborns, and you may see them around the nose. Caused by oil-secreting glands, the pimples may come and go during the first few days. You may also see petechia, red to purple pinpoints, on baby's face from the trauma of coming down the birth canal. These will disappear in a few days as well.

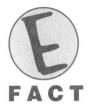

FACT

Your boy or girl may have swollen breasts that actually leak milk. This milk, known in folk medicine as "witch's milk," is the product of your pregnancy hormones at work on your newborn. Avoid massaging the area, as this can trigger an abscess. They will return to normal size within a few days.

The Umbilical Cord

Baby's umbilical cord stump looks just like it sounds, a dark, dried up protrusion. Since it is basically dead tissue, it is black in color. You'll be instructed to clean it regularly, usually with alcohol swabs, and keep it dry to prevent breakage and bleeding. Keep an eye open for signs of infection, such as pus or inflammation. Within 2 weeks or so, the stump will fall off and your baby's perfect little belly button will be revealed.

Genitals

Before your husband congratulates himself too heartily on your well-endowed son, you may want to break the news that it is probably just a passing phenomenon. Newborn boys and girls are often born with swollen genitals, again due to the effects of your pregnancy hormones working on them. Girls may even have a bit of mucus discharge, possibly blood-tinged, from their vaginas.

Fingernails and Toenails

Baby's tiny curled fingers and toes usually emerge in need of a manicure. Growing for several months in the womb, they are typically long and ragged. The thought of trimming such tiny appendages may fill you with dread, but it's not as hard as you might think. Just make sure you have the right tools (infant-sized clippers) and try to trim while baby is sleeping if you'd like to avoid wrestling with a moving target. If you still can't seem to get it down, bring your clippers with you to your 2-week pediatrician appointment and ask for pointers.

Sleeping Like a Baby

In the beginning, it will seem like your little one is sleeping quite a bit. In fact, she's snoozing up to 18 hours a day. If she's your first, you may be crouched outside her door waiting to run in and get some quality play time at the first rustle (second-time parents, on the other hand, count down the minutes to nap time). While her sleep patterns, which involve 4-hour stretches of snoozing, won't have a huge effect on your day schedule, they're going to hit you hard at night. She'll be waking up several times an evening for at least the first 3 months to be fed.

Remember to always place your baby on his back when laying him down for a nap or bedtime. Back sleeping has been shown to reduce the incidence of sudden infant death syndrome, or SIDS. Make sure baby's crib is clear of stuffed animals, quilts, pillows, and other soft bedding when he heads to bed as well.

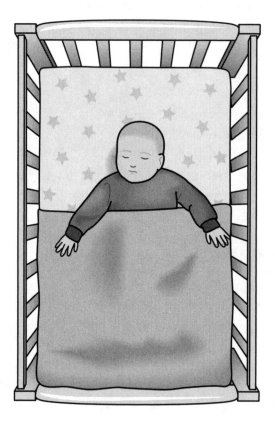

◄ Baby should always be put to sleep on his back. If a thin blanket is necessary, place baby with his feet at the bottom end of the crib and make sure the blanket is tucked in between mattress and crib and goes no higher than baby's chest.

Postpartum Depression

Feeling down is a common postpartum emotion that typically passes in a few weeks. For many women, however, these feelings go beyond the basic baby blues and signal a more serious depressive or endocrine disorder.

The Baby Blues

The majority of new mothers experience what has commonly become known as "the baby blues," a short-lived period of mild depression that appears in up to 85 percent of postpartum women. A severe shortage of sleep, disappointment with the birth experience, see-sawing hormone levels, anxieties about baby's health and well-being, and shaky confidence in your own parenting skills can all lead to feelings of sadness in inadequacy. Fortunately, most cases of the blues resolve themselves within a few days to 2 weeks after birth as balance returns to the new mother's life.

When It's More Than the Blues

More serious is postpartum depression (PPD), which occurs in about 10 percent of new mothers, and can drag on for up to a year. If you're experiencing one or more of the following symptoms, talk to your doctor about PPD:

- Feelings of extreme sadness and inexplicable crying jags
- Lack of pleasure in things you would normally enjoy
- Trouble concentrating
- Excessive worrying about the baby, or conversely, a lack of interest in the baby
- Feelings of low self-esteem
- Decreased appetite

Fortunately, PPD can be effectively treated with counseling and/or antidepressant drugs, so ask your doctor for a referral to a mental health professional. Even if you're breastfeeding, you may have medication options; there are several antidepressant drugs on the market that are thought to have minimal effects on nursing infants. A number of studies involving sertraline (Zoloft), for example, found that while the drug passes into breast milk, the levels it reaches in the nursing infant were clinically insignificant, in some cases too low to even be detected in standard laboratory blood tests.

Safety cannot be guaranteed, however; studies on how antidepressants might affect a breastfed child in the long term are not available. On the other hand, clinical research has demonstrated a measurable detrimental effect on children of depressed mothers when PPD goes untreated. Each woman must evaluate the risks of treatment versus the benefits when deciding if drug therapy is right for them.

Postpartum Psychosis

One in every 1,000 women experiences a severe form of PPD known as postpartum psychosis (or puerperal psychosis). Symptoms include hallucinations, delusions, contemplation of hurting oneself or others, insomnia, and turbulent mood swings. Postpartum psychosis is a medical emergency that needs immediate treatment and usually hospitalization. The good news is with proper medical care full recovery is expected.

Thyroid Problems

Thyroid problems are fairly common after childbirth, but the symptoms can be confused with other postpartum conditions. Milk supply difficulties, extreme fatigue, hair loss, depression, mood changes, problems losing weight or unusually rapid weight loss, heart palpitations, menstrual irregularities, and sleep disorders are all common signs of postpartum thyroid conditions.

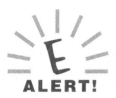

ALERT!

If you're experiencing signs of postpartum depression, make sure your doctor tests your thyroid levels. Up to 10 percent of new mothers experience thyroid problems following childbirth, and the symptoms of fatigue, depression, and unexplained weight loss can mimic postpartum depression.

Some women have temporary postpartum hyperthyroidism—an overactive thyroid, with weight loss, diarrhea, racing heart, anxiety, and other symptoms of a revved up metabolism. Doctors may prescribe drugs to ease symptoms, but this condition often resolves itself quickly.

Other women can develop temporary postpartum hypothyroidism—an underactive thyroid—with fatigue, weight gain, constipation, depression, and other symptoms of a slowed-down metabolism. Again, medication may be prescribed, depending on the severity of symptoms, and frequently the thyroid will return to normal within 6 months to a year after the birth.

New mothers with a family or personal history of autoimmune or thyroid disease may benefit from routine thyroid testing in the first month postpartum. It can be hard to tell what's "normal" after having a baby, but if any of the above symptoms become debilitating, a thyroid test can quickly rule out or diagnose a thyroid problem.

Women who experience temporary postpartum thyroid problems are at a higher risk to develop thyroid disease later in life, and should talk to their doctor about regular followup screening.

Adjusting to Your New Schedule

Many aspects of your life will be different now that you are a parent. You will probably feel that your priorities are very different now that you have a little one to think about. But taking time to care for yourself is equally important.

Bonding with Baby

These early weeks and months are a precious time of getting to know each other and building confidence. Yet as she's cried for 20 minutes straight and you still haven't guessed what's wrong (is she hungry, dirty, tired, colicky, gassy?) you may start to wonder about your mothering abilities. Trust yourself. It takes time to learn her language, but the patience and persistence you invest in decoding her signals will pay off. You'll crack the code eventually, and in the process you'll establish a bond of trust and communication that will last a lifetime.

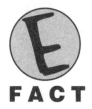

FACT

The term "bonding" was coined in 1976 by Drs. Marshall Klaus and John Kennell, two professors of pediatrics who published the pioneering work *Maternal-Infant Bonding.* Klaus and Kennell introduced the theory that close, personal contact between mother and baby was essential in the first 30 to 60 minutes after birth to build the foundation for a healthy attachment.

Sleep, or Lack of It

People told you how tired you would be when baby arrived, but after 3 months of uncomfortable and interrupted sleep leading up to the delivery, you thought you were well prepared. Surprise. You feel like the walking dead, and crave sleep constantly. Your baby will sleep through the night eventually. In the meantime, give yourself a break by splitting night duties with your spouse or significant others. Even if you're breastfeeding, if baby is in another room he can help out by retrieving and returning him. Also remember the new mom credo: "Nap when the baby naps." Forget laundry, forget dishes. You need your rest more than a clean house right now.

And if you've only slept 3 hours last night between bouts of calming a fussy baby? Don't get behind the wheel of a car before you get some adequate shuteye. Extreme fatigue slows your reaction time and you run a very real risk of falling asleep behind the wheel. The National Highway Traffic Safety Administration (NHTSA) estimates that driving while drowsy is responsible for at least 100,000 automobile accidents annually between the hours of 10 P.M. and 6 A.M.

Setting Priorities

You aren't going to be able to do it all. If you try to keep up your preparenthood schedule in addition to your new motherhood duties, something or someone has got to give. Usually it's your sanity. Things that just aren't that important, usually anything in the domesticity arena, can lag behind a bit. As the motivational gurus like to say, work smarter, not harder. Buy the birthday cake at the bakery instead of baking it yourself. Use a delivery service to get your groceries. Pay the kid down the block to mow the lawn.

Don't Forget to Have Fun

Once you get past the fatigue, the uncertainties, and the occasional frustrations, being a new mom can be incredibly entertaining. You have a legitimate excuse to play, explore, rhyme, sing, and revisit your childhood in general. You have an adoring little person who hangs on your every word and movement and loves you unconditionally. And you get to witness all her incredible firsts as your tiny miracle learns to smile, roll over, crawl, and eventually walk and talk. In a year, this postpartum time will be a distant memory. Treasure it while it's here.

The Rest of the Family

Obviously, you aren't doing this alone. Even if you're a single mom, you have people in your life who care for you and baby. Involve your family, or those around you, and baby and you will benefit.

Support

You might learn that your mother really does know a thing or two. It's amazing to watch her, and your dad, soothe and burp their grandchild like they were just doing it yesterday. Just like riding a bike, apparently, and they often have a baby wrangling trick or two up their sleeve that will make your life easier. Every family relationship is different, of course, but witnessing someone who raised you cuddle and care for the child that you will now nurture instills a sense of connectivity and completeness, as if your life has come full circle. Now just hope that all those prophecies they made about "hoping you have a child just like you" don't come to fruition!

Neighbors and friends will likely call to both check on the new addition and find out if they can do anything for you. One simple rule: Take all help that is offered. Don't feel guilty, don't feel like you're putting anyone out. They wouldn't offer if they didn't mean it. And if they offered just because they thought they should, they'll think twice next time won't they?

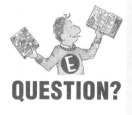

What's the best way to introduce a dog and new baby to each other?

Pets can be a wonderful influence in your child's life and create many happy memories, but only if they're properly supervised and trained. Because animals learn so much from scents, some new parents bring home a receiving blanket that smells like the new baby and give it to their dog to get acquainted. Let their first meeting be a gradual and calm affair with only immediate family present. And remember, even if you have the most mild mannered pet in the world, you need to preside over all his encounters with your child. It only takes a split second for baby to grasp a handful of fur and cause your pet to go on the defensive.

Sibling Rivalry

Give your older child a chance to bond with baby on the sibling level as well. Older kids frequently get a kick out of holding, feeding, and "protecting" their new little sister or brother. Children who are preschool age or younger may have a more difficult time accepting this drain on their parents' attention. Some tips to promote sibling harmony:

- If you're breastfeeding, establish a family routine of a snack or story when baby nurses to make it a special time for all.
- Involve your child in age-appropriate baby care. Helping with a bath or diaper change may be just the incentive they need to relish their new big brother or sister role.
- Try to arrange some special parental one-on-one time. Even if it's just a quick story during baby's nap, try to have a designated time where your firstborn is the star of the show.
- Tell your older child stories about their babyhood. Hearing how they threw strained peas at daddy or wore their very ripe diaper as a hat will have them in stitches and may help them relate to this odd little creature a bit better.
- Don't use the baby as an excuse. If they hear "We can't do that because the baby is sleeping" constantly, guess who they will start to

blame for the new crimp in their social life? Instead, provide baby-friendly alternatives when you say no: "We can't go swimming today, but we can go for a walk to the park." And arrange some time to take your "big kid" someplace he's been dying to go without a sibling in tow.

Daddy Time

Don't hog the baby. Make sure that daddy gets his own chance at bonding time. With a constant flow of visitors and your many hours clocked on baby duty, he may be feeling left out. Both he and your child need time alone together. Getting out and moving for a short walk is good exercise for you right now and a good way to clear your head after a day of talking in babyspeak. Hand the reins over, without direction or judgment if at all possible, and give dad a chance to run the show.

Just for Dads

Finally, a chance for hands-on parenting. Yet you may still find yourself feeling outside of the family circle. Are you hesitant to jump into this foreign world, or are you feeling like there isn't much left for you to handle? Remember that it is just as important for you to forge a strong bond with your child as it is for your significant other. Start small if it helps your confidence level. Even a task as simple as bundling your baby is an opportunity for relationship building.

Developing Your Own Daddy Style

There is more than one right way to change a diaper, warm a bottle, and calm a fussy baby. You will have your own way of doing things, and that is more than all right, that's good for your whole family. It teaches your baby that there are differences between mommy and daddy, and she will learn what to expect from your unique parenting style.

Don't be a bystander. If you feel like you're getting the brush-off when it comes to baby, let your partner know. She may be so preoccupied with new motherhood and other concerns that she isn't even aware she's doing it. Offer to take charge of regular tasks like bathing. If you feel a little shaky, ask mom to stay within shouting distance so you can get help if need be. But remember, the only reason she seems to handle baby so effortlessly is practice. That's all you need as well.

Set up a date for just baby and you—a trip to the park, a neighborhood walk, even some playtime in the backyard will do. Your partner can have some badly needed time to herself and you can stretch your caregiving wings.

Male Bonding

You are smitten, preoccupied, utterly in love with this new person in your life, and she with you. The feeling is aptly called engrossment, and it's your version of dad-to-baby bonding. Despite societal expectations and dated clichés of fatherhood, men can be just as nurturing and loving parents and caregivers as women. So dote on your child, spend time with her, play with her, diaper her, tickle her, and do anything else that comes naturally.

Easing Back into Intimacy

Once baby arrived and your wife got at least a shadow of her former self back, you thought sex would quickly follow. It hasn't. When you lay out the realities it shouldn't surprise you. Quick snatches of sleep, a sore and still recovering body, and all the concerns and anxieties that come with new motherhood are putting the damper on intimacy yet again.

If she is the primary caregiver at home with baby right now, there may be days when she doesn't even manage to get her clothes on until well past noon. Having dried spit up in your hair and baby poop on your pajama bottoms doesn't make you feel much like getting romantic. She needs a little empathy, TLC, and pampering (yes, again) to get back into a more amorous state of mind. Work on supporting her, helping with household duties, and encouraging her rest and recovery. Once her basic physical needs are met she can spend a little more time on the two of you.

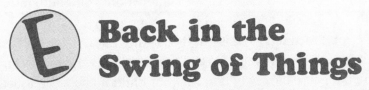

Chapter 21

Back in the Swing of Things

A lthough it seems overwhelming at first, it won't take you long to get the parenting basics down. Making career and family choices, building new and stronger relationships with your partner, and getting back in tune with your body are all priorities during the first year postpartum.

Getting Your Body Back

Another time-worn motherhood maxim that is worth repeating: It took 9 months for you to look this way, so give yourself at least that much time to get your body back. Actually, giving yourself a year is perhaps more realistic if you factor in a 3-month transitional period after the birth of your child. As you hammer out a routine where you and baby can manage to get dressed and bathed before dinnertime, you won't have much time for structured exercise in those early days.

Set realistic goals for weight loss. Losing weight too rapidly can actually be dangerous for you, and for your child if you're breastfeeding since you need 500 extra calories per day for nursing. In general, most women need to lose about 10 more pounds to return to their prepregnant weight at their 6-week postpartum visit. Many women find it difficult to lose weight during this period because they're working hard, nursing, and sleep-deprived. The time crunch all new mothers face can make a sensible and nutritious diet and regular exercise seem like a monumental task. Start slow and easy and the rest will follow.

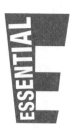

Stretch marks—your merit badges of pregnancy—are not going to disappear with exercise. If they haven't already, they will probably fade to barely noticeable silvery squiggles, and no one but you will probably even recognize them. But if you are self-conscious, studies have show that both Retin-A and laser treatment are effective methods for banishing them. Make an appointment with a dermatologist for further information, and if you're breastfeeding, be sure to let your doctor know so he can prescribe treatment and medications accordingly.

Exercise

Once you have your doctor's okay to get moving again, start slowly. Even if you were a fitness fanatic throughout pregnancy, you'll still have to ramp back up to reach your former conditioning level. Listen to your body. If you start experiencing bright red lochia discharge, it's a signal that you're probably doing too much, too fast.

If you've had a C-section, it's really important to stick to doctor's orders regarding exercise. Most providers will recommend at least a 6-week recovery time, but talk to your doctor about guidelines specific to you. Don't risk your health by starting a full-fledged campaign for your prepregnancy body before that time.

Many new moms find that their biggest challenge to regular exercise is just finding the time. Try these tips for squeezing it in:

- **Keep it simple.** Programs with steps, balls, bands, saucers, and other gear are probably not for you right now if you're just getting started. You haul around enough stuff just keeping baby clean and well fed. Don't add to it.
- **Baby steps.** Start small. Commit to 20 or 30 minutes a day of movement, and work your way up from there.
- **Pencil yourself in.** Set a regular schedule for your partner or a babysitter to care for baby, and use the time to get out and get moving.

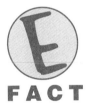

FACT

Many childhood education programs and community centers offer parent and child exercise classes, so check out this fun way to teach your child healthy fitness habits early on. If there are no classes in your neck of the woods, try one of the many kids' or child-parent exercise videos/DVDs on the market. Check your local library or movie rental shop first so you can find one you like before purchase.

- **Be flexible.** Do away with the all-or-nothing attitude. If you can't get to the gym one day, take a brisk walk or bike ride instead. Every little bit helps.
- **Buddy system.** If you're lucky enough to have a friend or neighbor nearby who is also a new mom, pair up. You can cheer each other on and commiserate.
- **Get baby in the act.** Get a jogging stroller and start a regular walking schedule, or simply incorporate more activity into your play. The park is a great place to start.

- **Join a gym.** Many health clubs and community programs (like the YMCA) have nursery areas for their members. This may be an option for you if financially feasible. Do take the opportunity to watch the staff in action before enrolling.

Eating Right

Exercise and good nutrition together are the best way to lose your pregnancy weight. If you established healthy eating patterns in pregnancy, you're ahead of the game. If not, now is as good a time as any to get started. Follow the food guide pyramid (see Chapter 1) and choose your foods wisely.

Breastfeeding shouldn't change your diet substantially. Some practitioners may advise a slight caloric increase of around 500 calories daily to meet milk production needs, but others believe no increase is necessary. You may also want to continue your daily prenatal vitamin. Talk to your doctor for specific guidance.

Another big benefit of breastfeeding can be a faster postpartum rate of weight loss. Although every mom is different, nursing helps you drop fat stores you collected in pregnancy for the very purpose of lactation. Your body works hard to produce milk, and also burns calories faster as a result.

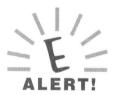

ALERT!

If you had gestational diabetes during your pregnancy, you have a higher risk of developing insulin resistance and type 2 diabetes. The American Diabetes Association recommends that your blood glucose levels be tested 6 weeks after pregnancy, and at subsequent three-year intervals thereafter (more frequently if you show signs of impaired glucose tolerance postpartum). Fortunately, lifestyle modifications such as exercise and weight loss are very effective at preventing of these conditions.

Typically, as long as you're choosing your foods wisely, you can let your stomach be your guide. Drink plenty of fluids. They're essential to keeping you well hydrated, and nursing has a tendency to make you thirsty. Having a glass of water or other noncaffeinated beverage each time baby nurses is a good ritual to establish proper fluid intake. The restrictions of pregnancy (no alcohol, tobacco, etc.) should also be continued throughout breastfeeding.

Making Up Sleep Deficits

Sleep is also an important factor in getting your old self back. If you're too tired to function, exercise has little appeal. You may find yourself opting for a fast food fix for dinner instead of taking the time and energy to prepare healthier fare. And your health can suffer as well. Sleep deprivation affects the immune system; chronic sleep loss has been linked to decreases in growth hormone (responsible for bone marrow growth and tissue healing); increased insulin resistance; and a decline in tumor necrosis factor (or natural killer cells; cancer and virus fighting agents). Mood disorders such as depression can also be made worse by insufficient sleep. And, of course, you're already aware of the zombie-like brain fog that those all-nighters bring. In short, sleep loss is a real health hazard. You can't run on empty forever.

So how do you get it back? Take naps whenever possible, of course, and consider a little creative shift work. If your child is not nursing when he wakes in the middle of the night, you can switch off night shift baby duty with dad so at least one of you has unbroken slumber every other day. This is even possible with breastfeeding if you've introduced a bottle to baby. Just pump breast milk the evening prior so your presence won't be necessary. You may get a protest the first time dad attempts to put baby back to sleep with a rubber nipple instead of mom's warm breast, but don't give up on the first try. Sometimes a little adjustment period is all that's necessary to ease into this new schedule.

The Incredible Changing Baby

Your infant will reach new milestones in such dizzying succession that you'll be convinced you have a prodigy on your hands. Watch her transform from a floppy-necked, bleary-eyed newborn to an active and alert infant in a matter of months. As she starts to become more aware of her surroundings, and interact more with you and her environment, providing encouragement, stimulation, and patience will help her to thrive.

Your pediatrician will give you an idea of appropriate developmental milestones as your baby grows. Remember, these are just averages, and some may be reached earlier and/or later than others. Every child grows at his own pace. The main function of milestones are to serve as a screening tool; if baby is lagging on many it may be a sign of a problem, but one or more delays are typically no cause for concern.

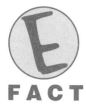

FACT

Preemie growth and development is assessed based on the age from estimated delivery date instead of actual birth date for the first 2 years of life. So a 4-month-old infant who was born one month prematurely would be assessed for her attainment of 3-month developmental milestones and size guidelines instead of 4-month milestones.

Your Career

As maternity leave approaches an end, you may find yourself faced with decisions you hadn't anticipated. The thought of leaving baby with a caregiver could be tearing you apart. Conversely, if you've put your career on hold for now to stay home with your child, you may find yourself missing the mental challenges and feelings of self-validation work provided. Changing your mind, either for or against a career outside the home, is not a terrible thing.

If You Decide Not to Return to Work

You had every intention of going back to the office after maternity leave was over, but you never expected to fall so deeply in love with not just your child, but motherhood. Or perhaps it's the thought of leaving your vulnerable little infant with someone outside of his immediate family that has you rethinking your options.

Financial concerns are an issue, of course. In many cases, the costs of child care and career-related expenses like dry cleaning bills and transportation costs can come close to offsetting the difference between a one- and two-income lifestyle. There may be a middle ground—picking up part-time work to cover the spread. Or, having dad stay home may be a viable alternative. Sit down and hash out the numbers with your partner. Flexibility, and creative thinking, may reveal a solution.

Going Back to Work

One of the hardest parts of new parenthood is heading back to the office. Getting up to speed on projects and procedures, handling the deluge from managers and coworkers who were basically lost without you, and fighting to stay off the "mommy track"—all while worrying about how your child is adapting to her new care arrangements—is a tall order to handle. If you can arrange it, try easing back into things with a reduced schedule (e.g., half days or 3 days a week) to smooth the transition for both of you. Chapter 9 has more information and advice on returning to work as a new mom, as well as breastfeeding basics for the office.

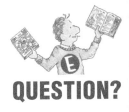

QUESTION?

How can I find good child care?
Your best source of leads for good child care is other moms in your life who share your values and viewpoints on child rearing. You can narrow down your list to facilities that have adequate staffing (for infants, this is generally a minimum of one provider to every three babies), a stimulating and child-friendly environment, and caring and nurturing staff. Proper licensing and accreditation are also important. The National Association for the Education of Young Children (NAEYC) has an online database of accredited providers and further advice on what to look for in a day care provider at ✑ *www.naeyc.org*.

Making Time for Yourself, and Using It

When your career gets back in the picture, things can accelerate to a frenzied pace. Don't just pay lip service to the idea of making time for yourself, do it. Even though it may be incredibly tempting to cancel your grown-up plans in favor of lazing around at home or getting some extra household chores covered, don't give in to the temptation. You'll find time alone, or with adult company (work doesn't count), is a great recharger. Here are some tips for following through.

- **Buy tickets to something.** You're less likely to bow out if there's money involved.
- **Invite a friend.** Again, committing to a date and event will make you more likely to follow through.
- **Pick something with a payoff.** A shopping trip to the one place where you know they have that hard-to-find Christmas gift you've been searching for may get you up and out.
- **Schedule a sitter right off the bat.** A short respite from child care, particularly if it leaves baby in the hands of a doting relative that would be sorely disappointed if you canceled, is a good incentive to keep your date with yourself.

A Whole New Family

Beyond your new parenting relationship, other family dynamics have definitely changed since baby's arrival. You and your partner may find yourselves hard pressed for time to spend together, and practical matters like money may be more of an issue as you learn how to adjust your lifestyle and income for three (or more). If you have some specific goals for family planning, you may even be thinking about pregnancy again.

Intimacy Issues

Perhaps for the first time in months, you may be rediscovering your interest in sex. Of course, your little one may be putting a damper on things unwittingly—rest assured she is bound to interrupt you in the height of passion at least once. Flexibility is key in having a healthy sex life with kids around. Grab time together when it presents itself, and follow these tips for rekindling the fire:

- **No baby talk.** Calling each other mommy and daddy around the kids is fine, but it can really kill the mood if it slips out in other circumstances.
- **Take it slow and easy.** Give both of you time to rediscover each other. There may be a learning curve with your post-pregnancy body.

- **Love yourself.** It's hard to enjoy lovemaking if you're self-conscious about the way you look. Accept the state of your body, whatever it is, and see it instead as a visible symbol of the miracle of your baby.
- **Quiet please.** You don't need to turn the baby monitor up to 11. Hearing every tiny baby sigh is a turnoff. Just turn the monitor down, or open your door instead; if she wakes up she will let you know.

Financial Planning

By now you've gotten a feel of how much it costs to care for your new family member, and you're either pleasantly surprised or in a panic. If it's the former, pat yourself on the back and consider saving your extra pennies in a new college fund for your child (a financial advisor can help you explore your options).

If you're in the panic category, take a deep breath and try to pinpoint the problem. Are the extra expenses coming from baby gadgetry and other nonessential purchases, or from necessities like diapers and wipes? A budget is really important in assessing the family finances now, so if you didn't create one during pregnancy, now is the time to start. There are places to cut back if you look for them. Finally, if you find yourself hopelessly in debt no matter how you look at the situation, you need to see a reputable credit counselor to get back on your financial footing. See Chapter 3 for more tips on money management.

The Next Time Around

The first birthday is usually about the time when everyone starts asking about a brother or sister for your "big"' kid. When you're done rolling your eyes and laughing, you start to actually give it some serious consideration. Are you ready to do it all over again?

Beyond physical readiness, how will you know? Suddenly, the sight of another woman in her ninth month brings about warm memories instead of enormous relief that it's someone else and not you, and you seem to have all but forgotten the perils of pregnancy and pain of childbirth.

If you're sold on a family with kids close enough in age to play and go to the same school together, you may be ready to start a bit sooner.

Try to give your body time to recover so that you don't cheat yourself and your next child out of a healthy pregnancy. A two-year breather from birth to birth is ideal.

Losing any excess pounds before starting over will make it easier for you to get through and beyond the next pregnancy. And take the same prepregnancy precautions with folic acid supplementation.

Just for Dads

Are you waiting for things to get back to normal? Stop right there. This is the new normal—take nothing for granted, be ready to change plans at a moment's notice, and learn to multitask. In other words, if you're a creature of habit and routine, you'll need to adjust your way of looking at the world.

The Night Shift

If you work a regular day job and then come home to play with and care for baby, it's easy to start burning the candle at both ends. You stay up later and later after baby's bedtime to get things done or just unwind, and end up only getting a few hours of sleep on the clock before she's up for another feeding. It's bad for your health and your sanity, so split the night shift with mom so you're at least getting all of your sleep half the time.

Making Adjustments

Life as a father is full of compromise. The library you and your wife had started is now a playroom, and the motorcycle you've been lusting after has been shelved (even with a sidecar, it just wouldn't be the same). You plan on spending your weekend watching the NFL draft, but reality strikes and you end up doing laps around the house with a sick and fussy baby instead. Yet instead of envying your childless friends who are at home awaiting the next pick, you look at your child and wish you could take the hurt away and be sick for her instead. Congratulations—you are a father.

Appendix A

Additional Resources

ABCs of Pregnancy—General Pregnancy Information

Reliable, comprehensive sources of pregnancy information and support.

About Pregnancy and Childbirth

With Robin Elise Weiss, L.C.C.E., I.C.C.E.-C.P.E., C.D. (D.O.N.A.)
✍ *http://pregnancy.about.com*

Ask Dr. Sears

With Dr. Bill Sears and Martha Sears, R.N.
✍ *www.askdrsears.org*

March of Dimes

Pregnancy and Newborn Health Education Center
✍ *www.marchofdimes.com*

The Visible Embryo

A pictorial tour of embryonic and fetal development created with a grant from the National Institutes of Health (NIH).
✍ *www.visembryo.com*

Childbirth Education

Find a childbirth educator or obtain more information on popular methods of childbirth (see also: "Professional Organizations," below).

The American Academy of Husband-Coached Childbirth

The Bradley Method
Box 5224
Sherman Oaks, CA 91413-5224
✆ 800-4-A-BIRTH
✍ *www.bradleybirth.org*

HypnoBirthing

P.O. Box 810
Epsom, NH 03234
E-mail: hypnobirthing@hypnobirthing.com
✍ *www.hypnobirthing.com*

Lamaze International

2025 M Street
Suite 800
Washington, DC 20036-3309
✆ 800-368-4404
✉ 202-367-2128
✍ *www.lamaze.org*

Marvelous Multiples

P.O. Box 381164
Birmingham, AL 35238
✆ 205-437-3575
✉ 205-437-3574
E-mail: marvmult@aol.com
✍ *www.marvelousmultiples.com*

Waterbirth International

Global Maternal/Child Health Association, Inc.
P.O. Box 1400
Wilsonville, OR 97070
✆ 800-641-2229
E-mail: info@waterbirth.org
✍ *www.waterbirth.org*

Complications in Pregnancy

Educational resources and support for complications in pregnancy.

About Diabetes

With Paula Ford-Martin

More information on the diagnosis and treatment of gestational diabetes.

✎ *http://diabetes.about.com*

Preeclampsia Foundation

P.O. Box 52993

Bellevue, WA 98015-2993

✆ 800-665-9341

E-mail: info@preeclampsia.org

✎ *www.preeclampsia.org*

Sidelines High-Risk Pregnancy Support National Office

P.O. Box 1808

Laguna Beach, CA 92652

✆ 888-447-4754 (HI-RISK4)

✎ 949-497-5598

E-mail: sidelines@sidelines.org

✎ *www.sidelines.org*

Having a Healthy Pregnancy

Resources for prenatal health.

About Stress Management

With Dr. Melissa Stöppler

✎ *http://stress.about.com*

Motherisk

The Hospital for Sick Children

555 University Avenue

Toronto, Ontario, Canada M5G 1X8
Alcohol and Substance Use Helpline: ✆ 877-327-4636
Nausea and Vomiting of Pregnancy Helpline: ✆ 800-436-8477
✎ *www.motherisk.org*

The National Toxicology Program (NTP)

Center for the Evaluation of Risks to Human Reproduction (CERHR)
NIEHS EC-32
P.O. Box 12233
Research Triangle Park, NC 27709
✆ 919-541-3455
✎ 919-316-4511
✎ *http://cerhr.niehs.nih.gov*

Infant Health and Development

Essentials for a healthy start in life.

Keep Kids Healthy

A Pediatrician's Guide to Your Children's Health and Safety
✎ *www.keepkidshealthy.com*

KidsHealth

A Project of the Nemours Foundation
✎ *www.kidshealth.org*

Zero to Three

National Center for Infants, Toddlers, and Families
2000 M Street, NW, Suite 200
Washington, DC 20036
✆ 202-638-1144
✎ *www.zerotothree.org*

Maternal and Infant Nutrition

Breastfeeding facts and support and nutrition assistance.

International Lactation Consultant Association

1500 Sunday Drive
Suite 102
Raleigh, NC 27607
✆ 919-787-5181
✍ *www.ilca.org*

La Leche League International

1400 N. Meacham Road
Schaumburg, IL 60173-4808
✆ 847-519-7730
✆ 1-800-LALECHE
✍ *www.lalecheleague.org*

Women, Infants, and Children (WIC)

Supplemental Food Programs Division
Food and Nutrition Service
United States Department of Agriculture
3101 Park Center Drive
Alexandria, VA 22302
✆ 703-305-2746
✇ 703-305-2196
✍ *www.fns.usda.gov/wic*

Postpartum Health Issues

Learn more about common maternal health issues occurring after birth.

About Thyroid Disease

With Mary Shomon
✍ *http://thyroid.about.com*
Find out more about postpartum thyroiditis.

Depression After Delivery

91 East Somerset Street
Raritan, NJ 08869
✆ 800-944-4773
✉ *www.depressionafterdelivery.com*

Professional Organizations

Need a referral? These professional organizations can help (see also: "Maternal and Infant Nutrition," page 328).

American College of Obstetricians and Gynecologists (ACOG)

Resource Center
409 12th Street S.W.
Washington, DC 20090-6920
✆ 202-863-2518
E-mail: resources@acog.org
✉ *www.acog.org*

American College of Nurse Midwives

818 Connecticut Avenue, NW
Suite 900
Washington, DC 20006
✆ 202-728-9860
✉ 202-728-9897
✉ *www.midwife.org*

Doulas of North America (DONA)

P.O. Box 626
Jasper, IN 47547
✆ 888-788-DONA
✉ 812-634-1491
E-mail: Referrals@dona.org
✉ *www.dona.org*

International Childbirth Education Association (ICEA)

P.O. Box 20048
Minneapolis, MN 55420
📞 952-854-8660
📠 952-854-8772
E-mail: info@icea.org
🖰 *www.icea.org*

National Association of Childbearing Centers (NACC)

3123 Gottschall Road
Perkiomenville, PA 18074
📞 215-234-8068
📠 215-234-8829
E-mail: ReachNACC@BirthCenters.org
🖰 *www.birthcenters.org*

National Society of Genetic Counselors (NSGC)

233 Canterbury Drive
Wallingford, PA 19086-6617
📞 610-872-7608
E-mail: nsgc@nsgc.org
🖰 *www.nsgc.org*

Special Issues

Special issues in pregnancy and beyond.

About Adoption

With Nancy Ashe
🖰 *http://adoption.about.com*

Hygeia Foundation for Perinatal Loss, Inc.

P.O. Box 3943   📞 203-387-3589
Amity Station   📠 203-387-3589
New Haven, CT 06525   🖰 *www.hygeia.org*

International Cesarean Awareness Network (ICAN)

1304 Kingsdale Avenue
Redondo Beach, CA 90278
✆ 310-542-6400
E-mail: info@ican-online.org
✎ *www.ican-online.org*

National Downs Syndrome Society (NDSS)

666 Broadway
New York, NY 10012
✆ 800-221-4602
✉ 212-979-2873
E-mail: info@ndss.org
✎ *www.ndss.org*

National Organization on Fetal Alcohol Syndrome (NOFAS)

216 G Street, North East
Washington, DC 20002
✆ 202-785-4585
✉ 202-466-6456
E-mail: information@nofas.org
✎ *www.nofas.org*

Spinal Bifida Association of America (SBAA)

4590 MacArthur Boulevard, NW
Suite 250
Washington, DC 20007-4226
✆ 800-621-3141 or ✆ 202-944-3285
✉ 202-944-3295
E-mail: sbaa@sbaa.org
✎ *www.sbaa.org*

VBAC.com

A "woman-centered, evidence based resource" on vaginal birth after
Caesarean section.
✎ *www.vbac.com*

Support for Single Mothers

Information and emotional support for unmarried mothers and moms-to-be.

Single Rose

Resources and forums for single moms.

www.singlerose.com

Single Parent Central

The "home of guerrilla single parenting" offers financial, career, and parenting information plus child support resources.

www.singleparentcentral.com

Twins or More

Resources for moms and dads of multiples (see also "Childbirth Education," above).

About Parenting Multiples

With Pamela Prindle Fierro

http://multiples.about.com

Mothers of Supertwins (MOST)

P.O. Box 951
Brentwood, NY 11717
631-859-1110
E-mail: info@MOSTonline.org
www.mostonline.org

National Organization of Mothers of Twins Clubs (NOMOTC)

Executive Office
P.O. Box 438
Thompson Station, TN 37179-0438
616-595-0936 or 800-243-2276
www.nomotc.org

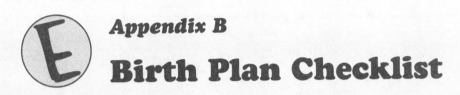

Appendix B

Birth Plan Checklist

Consider starting your birth plan with a short note to both your provider and the nursing staff who will be caring for you during labor and delivery. Explain your general wishes for a healthy and safe delivery, for joint decision-making should medical interventions be required, and for open communication throughout the process.

Read Chapter 15 to learn more about birth plans. Then use this checklist as a guide to assembling the basics.

1. Where will the birth take place?
   - ❑ Hospital
   - ❑ Birthing center
   - ❑ Home
   - ❑ Other: _____

2. Who will be there for labor support?
   - ❑ Husband or significant other
   - ❑ Doula
   - ❑ Friend
   - ❑ Family member

3. Will any room modifications or equipment be required to increase your comfort mentally and physically?
   - ❑ Objects from home (e.g., pictures, blanket, pillow)
   - ❑ Lighting adjustments
   - ❑ Music
   - ❑ Video or photos of birth
   - ❑ Other: _____

4. Any special requests for labor prep procedures?
   - ❑ Forego enema
   - ❑ Self-administer the enema
   - ❑ Forego shaving
   - ❑ Shave self
   - ❑ Heparin lock instead of routine IV line
   - ❑ Other: _____

5. Eating and drinking during labor?
   - ❏ Want access to a light snack
   - ❏ Want access to water, sports drink, or other appropriate beverage
   - ❏ Want ice chips
   - ❏ Other: _____

6. Do you want pain medication?
   - ❏ Analgesic (e.g., Stadol, Demerol, Nubain)
   - ❏ Epidural (if so, is timing an issue?)
   - ❏ Other: _____

7. What nonpharmaceutical pain relief equipment might you want access to?
   - ❏ Hydrotherapy (i.e., shower, whirlpool)
   - ❏ Warm compresses
   - ❏ Birth ball
   - ❏ Other: _____

8. What interventions would you like to avoid unless deemed a medical necessity by your provider during labor? Specify your preferred alternatives.
   - ❏ Episiotomy
   - ❏ Forceps
   - ❏ Internal fetal monitoring
   - ❏ Pitocin (oxytocin)
   - ❏ Other: _____

9. What would you like your first face-to-face with baby to be like?
   - ❏ Hold off on all nonessential treatment, evaluation, and tests for a specified time.
   - ❏ If immediate tests and evaluation is necessary, you, your partner, or another support person will accompany baby.
   - ❏ Want to nurse immediately following birth.
   - ❏ Would like family members to meet baby immediately following birth.
   - ❏ Other: _____

10. If a cesarean birth is required, what is important to you and your partner?
    - ❑ Type of anesthesia (e.g., general vs. spinal block)
    - ❑ Having partner or another support person present
    - ❑ Spending time with baby immediately following procedure
    - ❑ Bonding with baby in the recovery room
    - ❑ Type of postoperative pain relief and nursing considerations
    - ❑ Other: _____

11. Do you have a preference for who cuts the cord and when the cut is performed?
    - ❑ Mom
    - ❑ Dad
    - ❑ Provider
    - ❑ Delay until cord stops pulsing.
    - ❑ Cord blood will be banked. Cut per banking guidelines.
    - ❑ Cut at provider's discretion.
    - ❑ Other: _____

12. What kind of postpartum care will you and baby have at the hospital?
    - ❑ Baby will room-in with mom.
    - ❑ Baby will sleep in the nursery at night.
    - ❑ Baby will breastfeed.
    - ❑ Baby will bottle feed.
    - ❑ Baby will not be fed any supplemental formula and/or glucose water unless medically indicated.
    - ❑ Baby will not be given a pacifier.
    - ❑ Other: _____

13. Considerations for after discharge.
    - ❑ Support and short-term care for siblings
    - ❑ Support if you've had a caesarean
    - ❑ Maternity leave
    - ❑ Other: _____

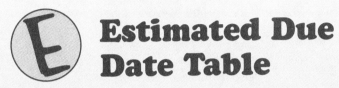

Appendix C

Estimated Due
Date Table

This chart lists due dates by month. Find the month and date on which your last menstrual period began, then look below that line to see what your estimated due date is.

| If your last period was... | 1/1 | 1/2 | 1/3 | 1/4 | 1/5 | 1/6 | 1/7 | 1/8 |
| Then your EDD is... | 10/8 | 10/9 | 10/10 | 10/11 | 10/12 | 10/13 | 10/14 | 10/15 |

| If your last period was... | 1/9 | 1/10 | 1/11 | 1/12 | 1/13 | 1/14 | 1/15 | 1/16 |
| Then your EDD is... | 10/16 | 10/17 | 10/18 | 10/19 | 10/20 | 10/21 | 10/22 | 10/23 |

| If your last period was... | 1/17 | 1/18 | 1/19 | 1/20 | 1/21 | 1/22 | 1/23 | 1/24 |
| Then your EDD is... | 10/24 | 10/25 | 10/26 | 10/27 | 10/28 | 10/29 | 10/30 | 10/31 |

| If your last period was... | 1/25 | 1/26 | 1/27 | 1/28 | 1/29 | 1/30 | 1/31 | |
| Then your EDD is... | 11/1 | 11/2 | 11/3 | 11/4 | 11/5 | 11/6 | 11/7 | |

| If your last period was... | 2/1 | 2/2 | 2/3 | 2/4 | 2/5 | 2/6 | 2/7 | 2/8 |
| Then your EDD is... | 11/8 | 11/9 | 11/10 | 11/11 | 11/12 | 11/13 | 11/14 | 11/15 |

| If your last period was... | 2/9 | 2/10 | 2/11 | 2/12 | 2/13 | 2/14 | 2/15 | 2/16 |
| Then your EDD is... | 11/16 | 11/17 | 11/18 | 11/19 | 11/20 | 11/21 | 11/22 | 11/23 |

| If your last period was... | 2/17 | 2/18 | 2/19 | 2/20 | 2/21 | 2/22 | 2/23 | 2/24 |
| Then your EDD is... | 11/24 | 11/25 | 11/26 | 11/27 | 11/28 | 11/29 | 11/30 | 12/1 |

| If your last period was... | 2/25 | 2/26 | 2/27 | 2/28 | | | | |
| Then your EDD is... | 12/2 | 12/3 | 12/4 | 12/5 | | | | |

| If your last period was... | 3/1 | 3/2 | 3/3 | 3/4 | 3/5 | 3/6 | 3/7 | 3/8 |
| Then your EDD is... | 12/6 | 12/7 | 12/8 | 12/9 | 12/10 | 12/11 | 12/12 | 12/13 |

| If your last period was... | 3/9 | 3/10 | 3/11 | 3/12 | 3/13 | 3/14 | 3/15 | 3/16 |
| Then your EDD is... | 12/14 | 12/15 | 12/16 | 12/17 | 12/18 | 12/19 | 12/20 | 12/21 |

| If your last period was... | 3/17 | 3/18 | 3/19 | 3/20 | 3/21 | 3/22 | 3/23 | 3/24 |
| Then your EDD is... | 12/22 | 12/23 | 12/24 | 12/25 | 12/26 | 12/27 | 12/28 | 12/29 |

| If your last period was... | 3/25 | 3/26 | 3/27 | 3/28 | 3/29 | 3/30 | 3/31 | |
| Then your EDD is... | 12/30 | 12/31 | 1/1 | 1/2 | 1/3 | 1/4 | 1/5 | |

| If your last period was... | 4/1 | 4/2 | 4/3 | 4/4 | 4/5 | 4/6 | 4/7 | 4/8 |
| Then your EDD is... | 1/6 | 1/7 | 1/8 | 1/9 | 1/10 | 1/11 | 1/12 | 1/13 |

| If your last period was... | 4/9 | 4/10 | 4/11 | 4/12 | 4/13 | 4/14 | 4/15 | 4/16 |
| Then your EDD is... | 1/14 | 1/15 | 1/16 | 1/17 | 1/18 | 1/19 | 1/20 | 1/21 |

| If your last period was... | 4/17 | 4/18 | 4/19 | 4/20 | 4/21 | 4/22 | 4/23 | 4/24 |
| Then your EDD is... | 1/22 | 1/23 | 1/24 | 1/25 | 1/26 | 1/27 | 1/28 | 1/29 |

| If your last period was... | 4/25 | 4/26 | 4/27 | 4/28 | 4/29 | 4/30 | | |
| Then your EDD is... | 1/30 | 1/31 | 2/1 | 2/2 | 2/3 | 2/4 | | |

| If your last period was... | 5/1 | 5/2 | 5/3 | 5/4 | 5/5 | 5/6 | 5/7 | 5/8 |
| Then your EDD is... | 2/5 | 2/6 | 2/7 | 2/8 | 2/9 | 2/10 | 2/11 | 2/12 |

| If your last period was... | 5/9 | 5/10 | 5/11 | 5/12 | 5/13 | 5/14 | 5/15 | 5/16 |
| Then your EDD is... | 2/13 | 2/14 | 2/15 | 2/16 | 2/17 | 2/18 | 2/19 | 2/20 |

| If your last period was... | 5/17 | 5/18 | 5/19 | 5/20 | 5/21 | 5/22 | 5/23 | 5/24 |
| Then your EDD is... | 2/21 | 2/22 | 2/23 | 2/24 | 2/25 | 2/26 | 2/27 | 2/28 |

| If your last period was... | 5/25 | 5/26 | 5/27 | 5/28 | 5/29 | 5/30 | 5/31 | |
| Then your EDD is... | 3/1 | 3/2 | 3/3 | 3/4 | 3/5 | 3/6 | 3/7 | |

| If your last period was... | 6/1 | 6/2 | 6/3 | 6/4 | 6/5 | 6/6 | 6/7 | 6/8 |
| Then your EDD is... | 3/8 | 3/9 | 3/10 | 3/11 | 3/12 | 3/13 | 3/14 | 3/15 |

| If your last period was... | 6/9 | 6/10 | 6/11 | 6/12 | 6/13 | 6/14 | 6/15 | 6/16 |
| Then your EDD is... | 3/16 | 3/17 | 3/18 | 3/19 | 3/20 | 3/21 | 3/22 | 3/23 |

| If your last period was... | 6/17 | 6/18 | 6/19 | 6/20 | 6/21 | 6/22 | 6/23 | 6/24 |
| Then your EDD is... | 3/24 | 3/25 | 3/26 | 3/27 | 3/28 | 3/29 | 3/30 | 3/31 |

| If your last period was... | 6/25 | 6/26 | 6/27 | 6/28 | 6/29 | 6/30 | | |
| Then your EDD is... | 4/1 | 4/2 | 4/3 | 4/4 | 4/5 | 4/6 | | |

| If your last period was... | 7/1 | 7/2 | 7/3 | 7/4 | 7/5 | 7/6 | 7/7 | 7/8 |
| Then your EDD is... | 4/7 | 4/8 | 4/9 | 4/10 | 4/11 | 4/12 | 4/13 | 4/14 |

| If your last period was... | 7/9 | 7/10 | 7/11 | 7/12 | 7/13 | 7/14 | 7/15 | 7/16 |
| Then your EDD is... | 4/15 | 4/16 | 4/17 | 4/18 | 4/19 | 4/20 | 4/21 | 4/22 |

| If your last period was... | 7/17 | 7/18 | 7/19 | 7/20 | 7/21 | 7/22 | 7/23 | 7/24 |
| Then your EDD is... | 4/23 | 4/24 | 4/25 | 4/26 | 4/27 | 4/28 | 4/29 | 4/30 |

| If your last period was... | 7/5 | 7/26 | 7/27 | 7/28 | 7/29 | 7/30 | 7/31 | |
| Then your EDD is... | 5/1 | 5/2 | 5/3 | 5/4 | 5/5 | 5/6 | 5/7 | |

| If your last period was... | 8/1 | 8/2 | 8/3 | 8/4 | 8/5 | 8/6 | 8/7 | 8/8 |
| Then your EDD is... | 5/8 | 5/9 | 5/10 | 5/11 | 5/12 | 5/13 | 5/14 | 5/15 |

| If your last period was... | 8/9 | 8/10 | 8/11 | 8/12 | 8/13 | 8/14 | 8/15 | 8/16 |
| Then your EDD is... | 5/16 | 5/17 | 5/18 | 5/19 | 5/20 | 5/21 | 5/22 | 5/23 |

| If your last period was... | 8/17 | 8/18 | 8/19 | 8/20 | 8/21 | 8/22 | 8/23 | 8/24 |
| Then your EDD is... | 5/24 | 5/25 | 5/26 | 5/27 | 5/28 | 5/29 | 5/30 | 5/31 |

| If your last period was... | 8/25 | 8/26 | 8/27 | 8/28 | 8/29 | 8/30 | 8/31 | |
| Then your EDD is... | 6/1 | 6/2 | 6/3 | 6/4 | 6/5 | 6/6 | 6/7 | |

If your last period was...	9/1	9/2	9/3	9/4	9/5	9/6	9/7	9/8
Then your EDD is...	6/8	6/9	6/10	6/11	6/12	6/13	6/14	6/15

If your last period was...	9/9	9/10	9/11	9/12	9/13	9/14	9/15	9/16
Then your EDD is...	6/16	6/17	6/18	6/19	6/20	6/21	6/22	6/23

If your last period was...	9/17	9/18	9/19	9/20	9/21	9/22	9/23	9/24
Then your EDD is...	6/24	6/25	6/26	6/27	6/28	6/29	6/30	7/1

If your last period was...	9/25	9/26	9/27	9/28	9/29	9/30		
Then your EDD is...	7/2	7/3	7/4	7/5	7/6	7/7		

If your last period was...	10/1	10/2	10/3	10/4	10/5	10/6	10/7	10/8
Then your EDD is...	7/8	7/9	7/10	7/11	7/12	7/13	7/14	7/15

If your last period was...	10/9	10/10	10/11	10/12	10/13	10/14	10/15	10/16
Then your EDD is...	7/16	7/17	7/18	7/19	7/20	7/21	7/22	7/23

If your last period was...	10/17	10/18	10/19	10/20	10/21	10/22	10/23	10/24
Then your EDD is...	7/24	7/5	7/26	7/27	7/28	7/29	7/30	7/31

If your last period was...	10/25	10/26	10/27	10/28	10/29	10/30	10/31	
Then your EDD is...	8/1	8/2	8/3	8/4	8/5	8/6	8/7	

If your last period was...	11/1	11/2	11/3	11/4	11/5	11/6	11/7	11/8
Then your EDD is...	8/8	8/9	8/10	8/11	8/12	8/13	8/14	8/15

If your last period was...	11/9	11/10	11/11	11/12	11/13	11/14	11/15	11/16
Then your EDD is...	8/16	8/17	8/18	8/19	8/20	8/21	8/22	8/23

If your last period was...	11/17	11/18	11/19	11/20	11/21	11/22	11/23	11/24
Then your EDD is...	8/24	8/25	8/26	8/27	8/28	8/29	8/30	8/31

If your last period was...	11/25	11/26	11/27	11/28	11/29	11/30		
Then your EDD is...	9/1	9/2	9/3	9/4	9/5	9/6		

If your last period was...	12/1	12/2	12/3	12/4	12/5	12/6	12/7	12/8
Then your EDD is...	9/7	9/8	9/9	9/10	9/11	9/12	9/13	9/14

If your last period was...	12/9	12/10	12/11	12/12	12/13	12/14	12/15	12/16
Then your EDD is...	9/15	9/16	9/17	9/18	9/19	9/20	9/21	9/22

If your last period was...	12/17	12/18	12/19	12/20	12/21	12/22	12/23	12/24
Then your EDD is...	9/23	9/24	9/25	9/26	9/27	9/28	9/29	9/30

If your last period was...	12/25	12/26	12/27	12/28	12/29	12/30	12/31	
Then your EDD is...	10/1	10/2	10/3	10/4	10/5	10/6	10/7	

Appendix D

The Practical Side of Pregnancy— A 9-Month Checklist

Your health care provider will keep you abreast of what medical steps you should be taking throughout your pregnancy, but there are plenty of practical matters you and your partner will need to address that aren't covered by doctor's orders. This month-by-month checklist provides a handy reference list to make sure you've covered the basics. Rearrange the timeline to your own schedule and pregnancy, if needed, and turn to the referenced chapters for further details and tips on each item.

Month 1

- ❑ Evaluate your doctor or group practice and decide if it's right for you and your pregnancy. (Chapter 1)
- ❑ Get up to speed on your health insurance coverage for prenatal visits, delivery, and the care of your child. (Chapter 3)
- ❑ If you smoke or drink, quit now. (Chapter 1)
- ❑ Discuss any possible on-the-job hazards with your physician. (Chapter 9)

Month 2

- ❑ Start developing a maternity wardrobe. (Chapter 4)
- ❑ Take inventory of what baby or maternity items you will "inherit" from friends and family. (Chapter 4)
- ❑ Share the good news with your other kids. (Chapter 11)
- ❑ Sit down with your partner and start working out a post-baby budget. (Chapter 3)

Month 3

- ❑ Inform your employer. (Chapters 6 and 9)
- ❑ Get details on your maternity benefits. (Chapter 9)
- ❑ Look into a prenatal exercise class. (Chapter 8)
- ❑ Decide where the baby's room or space will be. (Chapter 3)
- ❑ Make sleep a priority; set a new early bedtime and stick to it. (Chapter 10)

Month 4

❑ Treat yourself and your kids to a special day out. (Chapters 11 and 12)

❑ Compare and decide on cloth versus disposable diapers. (Chapter 16)

❑ Find out how and when to add your new baby to your insurance coverage. (Chapter 3)

❑ If you don't have one, shop for a crib that meets current safety standards. (Chapter 3)

❑ Do some basic babyproofing. (Chapter 3)

Month 5

❑ Plan a special night out with your partner. (Chapter 12)

❑ Perform a pre-baby car check. (Chapter 3)

- Ensure that your vehicle is child-seat friendly.
- Purchase a rear-facing infant seat for your child.
- Try your hand at properly installing it in your vehicle.

❑ Explore child care options for your new baby. (Chapters 9 and 21)

Month 6

❑ Take a day off and pamper yourself. (Chapter 12)

❑ Start putting together your birth plan. (Chapter 15)

❑ Think about who you want in the delivery room. (Chapter 15)

❑ Contemplate the breast versus bottle decision. (Chapter 19)

❑ Discuss your maternity leave plans with your employer. (Chapter 9)

Month 7

❑ Make a date with yourself to relax, read, or just catch up on sleep. (Chapter 12)

❑ Interview pediatricians. (Chapter 14)

❑ Sign up for childbirth classes. (Chapter 14)

❑ Sign your child up for sibling classes. (Chapters 11 and 14)

❑ Set up an appointment to discuss your birth plan with your provider. (Chapter 15)

❑ Arrange for care for your other children during your hospital stay. (Chapter 17)

Month 8

❑ Take five and de-stress; it's good for you and baby. (Chapter 4)

❑ Prepare baby's room or sleep space. (Chapter 3)

❑ Lay out your baby essentials. (Chapter 16)

❑ Discuss circumcision with your pediatrician and your partner. (Chapter 18)

❑ Start wrapping up projects at work. (Chapter 9)

❑ Finalize your child care plans for after maternity leave. (Chapters 9 and 21)

❑ Preregister at your hospital or birthing center. (Chapter 15)

Month 9

❑ Make sure that your other children's teachers and care providers are aware of your impending hospital stay. (Chapter 17)

❑ Pack your bag and compile a call list for your partner. (Chapter 17)

❑ Line up postpartum assistance. (Chapter 17)

❑ Stock up the freezer with heat-and-eat meals, or recruit postpartum kitchen help. (Chapter 17)

❑ Make a plan, and a backup plan, for getting to the hospital. (Chapter 17)

❑ Put your feet up, relax, and take a deep breath—the rest is up to baby!

Index

A

Abdominal pain, 32, 122, 144, 182, 192, 194, 195, 198
Activities, restricted, 122
Afterpains, 298
Age, and risks, 20
Air embolism, 175
Airline travel, 231
Albumin, 69
Alcohol consumption, *x*, 10–11, 317
Alcohol-related developmental disabilities (ARDD), 11
Alpha-fetoprotein (AFP) blood tests, 74, 78–79, 90, 101, 119, 181
American Academy of Pediatrics, 285
American Association of Pediatrics, 270
American Board of Genetic Counseling, 20
American College of Nurse Midwives, 6
American College of Obstetrics and Gynecology (ACOG), 3–4, 6, 15
American Diabetes Association, 72, 316
American Dietetic Association, 289
Amniocentesis, 56, 74, 79–81, 104, 180, 181
Amnion, 24, 25
Amniotic fluid, 25, 56, 84
Amniotic fluid, leaking, 195, 197, 199, 205, 229, 242
Amniotic sac, 25
Amniotomy, 265
Analgesics, 255
Anemia, 12, 71, 73, 103, 181, 231
Anencephaly, 12–13
Anesthetics, 255–57, 263
Ankles, swelling of, 122, 169–70, 193
Antacids, 117
Antepartum depression, 19
Antibiotics, 17
Antiemetics, 37

Anxieties, 34, 38, 236–37, 244
Apgar test, 267
Apgar, Virginia, 267
Appendicitis, 187
Aspartame, 174
Aspirin, 18
Assisted reproductive technology (ART), 99, 100
Asthma, 21

B

Baby
    anatomy of, 301–3
    bathing, 238
    birth of, 260–61, 266–67
    bonding with, 307–8
    bringing home, 297–312
    burping, 286, *287–88*
    cost of, 45–50, 96
    crib for, 40, 41
    development of, 25, *26*, 55–56, *57*, 86, *87*, *114*, 114–15, *142*, 142–43, *168*, 168–69, *202*, 202–3, *228*, 228–29, 240–41
    diaper changes, 237–38
    doctor visits, 267
    dropping down, 241
    due date, *x*, 30–31, 242, 248–49, 337–40
    fingernails, 303
    first bowel movement, 197
    gender of, 56, 78, 86
    genitals, 303
    growth of, 317–18
    heartbeat of, 82–84, 90–91, 119
    hunger signs, 291
    measuring, 90
    meeting, 266–67
    movements of, 56, 118, 147
    names for, 95, 237
    overdue baby, 248–49
    in parent's room, 40, 235
    preparing for, 40–51, 235–36

    reflexes of, 300
    safety issues, 40–41, 44–45
    size of, 240
    skin of, 302–3
    sleep positions for, 40, 304
    soft spot, 291, 301, 302
    space for, 40–41, 235
    supplies for, 47–49, 235–36
    testing, 267
    toenails, 303
    weight gain, 291
    weight loss, 300
    see also Fetus
"Baby blues," 305
Baby-proofing home, 41, 44–45
Babysitters, 48, 136. *See also* Child care
Back pain, 144, 195, 199, 241, 254
Bargain hunting, 47–48
Bed rest, 196–98
Beer, 10–11
Belly form, 63
Belly support band, 147
Bing classes, 147
Biochemical balance, 18–19
Biophysical profile (BPP), 83, 84
Birth ball, 223
Birth control, 299
Birth defects
    causes of, 10, 12, 15, 17–18, 73
    history of, 19–20
    testing for, 57, 73, 74
Birth of baby, 260–61, 266–67
Birth plan
    benefits of, *x*
    creating, 206–7, 215–26, 333–36
    finalizing, 245
    flexibility in, 217, 223–24
    presenting to doctor, 7, 216–17
Birth weight, 9, 61, 71, 92
Birth Without Violence, 209
Birthing centers
    arriving on-time, 234
    atmosphere of, 218–19

childbirth classes, 210
packing for stay, 245–47
policies of, 6–7, 225
preregistration, 220
stay in, 268–69
touring, 210
visitors, 219–20, 268–69
Blastocyst, 24
Blended families, 159
Blood clot, 171
Blood pressure, 68, 70
Blood type, 72
Bonding, 40, 108, 307–8, 311, 312
Botanical substances, 18, 36
Bottle feeding, 112, 226, 236, 277–78, 286
Bradley classes, 147, 209, 324
Bradley, Robert, 209
Braxton-Hicks contractions, 204, 242
Breastfeeding
benefits of, 48, 110, 278, 279, 285
birth plan for, 226
bras for, 203–4, 284–85
caloric recommendations, 289
classes for, 207
finger feeding, 295
in hospital, 226, 246, 267, 269
lactation consultants, 269, 293
lactation facilities, 130, 137, 139
lactation problems, 291–95
latching on, 280
letdown, 284
milk supply, 291–92
multiples, 109–12
positions, 110–12, 280, 281–83
pros and cons, 276–77
in public, 290
pumping milk, 278, 294
schedules, 284, 285, 291
and stress, 292
supplementing, 294
support for, 291, 295–96
techniques, 280–84
and work, 137, 139, 278

Breasts
changes in, 26
engorgement, 269, 279, 299
leaking, 203
mastitis, 295
tenderness of, 26, 59, 203, 269, 279, 299
Breath, shortness of, 122
Breech birth, 106, 231–32, 262
Bronchopulmonary dysplasia (BPD), 107
Budgets, 48–49

C

Calcium, 31, 117
Caloric recommendations, 11, 87, 102, 229, 289, 314
Cancer, 184, 188
Car seats, 41–42, 43
Cardiovascular system, 27–28
Career, and family, x, 125–40, 248, 278, 318–19
Carrying during pregnancy, 119, 241
Catheter, 256, 263
Cats, 59
Caudal block, 257
Centers for Disease Control (CDC), 11, 243, 266
Central nervous system (CNS), 10, 11
Cerclage, 103, 188
Cerebral palsy, 105
Cervical incompetence, 187–88, 196
Cervical length, 103
Cervical ripening, 68, 241, 243, 258, 265–66
Cesarean section
anesthetics, 255, 256, 263
birth plan for, 210, 224
for breech births, 231
cost of, 45
epidurals, 256, 257
exercise after, 315
for multiple births, 102, 106
planning, 148
process of, 262–65

recovery from, 247, 268, 269, 299
with second pregnancy, 156, 210
stress tests, 84
support during, 271
Chest pain, 122
Chickenpox, 73, 119
Child care, 48, 136, 138, 319
Childbirth, 224, 260–61, 266–67, 272–73
Childbirth classes, 147–48, 207–13
Childbirth education, 324–25
Childbirth options
birthing rooms, 218–19
cutting cord, 224
following birth, 225
natural childbirth, 209, 223
visitors, 219–20, 268–69
Childbirth Without Fear, 209
Children
classes for, 211
cost of raising, 48, 50, 96
involving, 162–63
with new baby, 158–63
regressions, 162
time with, 174–75
see also Siblings
Chills, 33
Chlamydia, 75
Chloasma, 58
Choriocarcinoma, 184
Chorion, 24, 25
Chorionic villus sampling (CVS), 57, 74, 81–82, 181
Choroid plexus cysts, 182
Chromosomal abnormalities, 57, 78, 80–82, 90, 180, 182–83
Chromosomes, 180
Chronic health problems, 21, 180
Circumcision, 270
Clear cell adenocarcinoma, 188
Colostrum, 203, 269, 279
Conception, 24, 30
Confirming pregnancy, 30
Congenital abnormalities, 62, 106
Congestion, 34, 59, 151
Constipation, 27–28, 89, 117, 298–99

Consumer Product Safety Commission, 44
Contraception, 299
Contraction stress test (CST), 84
Contractions
    Braxton-Hicks contractions, 204, 242
    increase in, 242
    intervals between, 242, 252, 258
    monitoring, 82–83, 221
    painful contractions, 204–5
    preterm labor, 103–4
    stopping, 104
Corticosteroids, 196
Corticotropin-releasing hormone (CRH), 61
Cortisol, 19
Costs
    of baby, 45–50, 96
    of Cesarean section, 45
    of delivery, 6, 45
    of health insurance, 49
    of raising children, 48, 50, 96
Couple time, 175, 176, 320–21
Coupon clubs, 47
Couvade, 52
Cramping, 32, 192, 195, 198
Cramping, of legs, 170–71
Cribs, 40, 41
CT scans, 128, 129
Cystic fibrosis, 73, 181

D

Dads
    anxieties, 236–37
    bathing baby, 238
    bonding with baby, 311, 312
    bottle feeding, 296
    breastfeeding support, 295–96
    checklist for, 249
    classes for, 212–13, 237
    as coach, 213, 258, 259, 260, 270–71
    compromises, 322
    diaper duties, 237–38
    education, 152–53
    fatherhood, 237, 311–12, 322

handling stress, 177
    help from, 123–24
    hospital trip, 249–50
    paternity leave, 126, 127, 134, 138
    pregnancy symptoms, 52, 66
    responsibilities of, 96, 153, 311–12
    role of, 38, 95–96, 123–24, 249–50
    second pregnancies, 163–64
    sharing pregnancy with, 51–52, 176–77
    see also Partner; Spouse
Day care. See Child care
Deep vein thrombosis (DVT), 171
Delivery
    complications during, 272–73
    cost of, 45
    estimated date of, x, 30–31, 242, 248–49, 337–40
    medical interventions, 6
    moment of, 260–61
    of multiples, 101–2, 106–8
    responsibility of, 6
Depression, 19, 305–7
Developmental problems, 10
Diabetes
    gestational diabetes, 69, 70, 71, 90, 172, 184–87, 316
    risks, 20, 186–87, 231
    treatment for, 21, 185
    types of, 180, 316
Diabetic ketoacidosis (DKA), 69
Diagnostic tests, 29, 60, 67, 243
Diapers, 48–49, 236–38, 291
Diarrhea, 33
Dick-Read, Grantly, 209
Diet, 11–15, 88, 289, 316
Diethylstilbestrol, 187, 188, 195
Dilation, 103, 187–88, 196, 243, 258–61
Dilation and curettage (D & C), 183
Discrimination, x, 126–27
Dizygotic twins, 98, 99
Dizziness, 28, 59, 122, 182
DNA testing, 180
Doctors
    communication skills, 7–8
    first visits, 28–29

gender of, 8
    importance of, xii
    interviewing, 6–7
    personality of, 8
    selecting, 4–8
    visits when working, 133
    visits with, 4, 28–33, 59–60, 68, 90–91, 101–2, 147–48, 172, 205–6, 231, 242
Doula, 4, 53, 220
Down syndrome, 20, 78, 80, 181
Dreams, 120
"Dropping down," 241, 242
Drugs, 16
Dry mouth, 221
Due date, x, 30–31, 242, 248–49, 337–40

E

Eclampsia, 193–94
Ectopic pregnancy, 181–82, 187, 188
Edema, 170, 230
Edwards syndrome, 182
Eighth month, 227–38
Electrical outlets, 44
Electrolyte balance, 37, 187
Embryo, 23–25, 26
Emergency phone calls, 7, 32–33
Emotions
    in first trimester, 33–34, 51–52, 60–62
    following birth, 266–67
    in second trimester, 123–24, 148–49
    in third trimester, 234, 243–44
Employment issues, 125–40, 248, 278, 318–19
Endometriosis, 181
Endometrium, 24
Engagement, 241
Environmental Protection Agency (EPA), 44
Epidural, 223, 256, 257, 263
Episiotomy, 223, 261, 262, 268
Estimated date of delivery (EDD), x, 30–31, 242, 248–49, 337–40

Estradiol, 58
Estriol, 78
Ethnic heritage, 2
Examinations, 32
Excitement, 33, 236–37
Exercise
   after birth, 314–16
   benefits of, 15, 120–22
   flexibility exercises, 146
   Kegel exercises, 122, 229
   off-limit activities, 15, 122
   pelvic tilt exercises, 144, *145*
   precautions, 122
   and stress, 62
External cephalic version, 231, 232

F

Face, swelling of, 170
Facial anomalies, 10, 11
Faintness, 28, 59
Faith issues, 54
Fallopian tube, 24
Fallopian tube pregnancy, 181–82
False alarms, 250
Family
   assistance from, 247, 309
   background of, 2–3, 20
   and career, *x*, 125–40, 248, 278,
      318–19
   sharing pregnancy with, 54
Family-friendly companies, 137–38
Family leave plan, 94–95, 126–27
Family matters, 39–54
Family Medical Leave Act (FMLA),
   127, 134
Family planning, 164–65, 299, 320–22
Fatherhood. *See* Dads
Fatigue, 27, 59
Feeding schedules, 284, 285
Feet, swelling of, 122, 169–70, 193
Fertility treatments, 99, 100
Fertilization, 23, 24, *98*
Fetal alcohol effects (FAE), 11
Fetal alcohol syndrome
   (FAS), 10, 11

Fetal heart rate (FHR), 82–84,
   90–91, 119, 221, 253, 256
Fetal macrosomia, 186, 249
Fetal movements, counting, 147, 241
Fetal sleep cycle, 150
Fetus
   development of, 25, *26*, 55–56,
      57, 86, *87*, *114*, 114–15
   size of, 25, 56, 86, 114, 142, 168,
      202, 228, 240
   see also Baby
Fever, 33, 144, 199
Fiber, 89, 117, 299
Fifth month, 141–53
Financial aid programs, 46, 53
Financial planning, 48–50, 321
First month, 23–38
First-time parents, 51
First trimester
   alcohol consumption during, 11
   development of embryo, 24–25
   emotions during, 33–34, 51–52, 60–62
   exercise during, 15
   hormonal changes during, 25–28
   length of, 23
   smoking during, 9–10
   symptoms during, 27–28, 59, 89,
      91–92, 100–101
   weight gain, 58, 87
Fluid leakage. *See* Amniotic fluid
Fluids, drinking, 36, 37, 102, 117, 221,
   289, 299, 316
Fluttering, 56, 118
Flying, 231
Folate, 12–13
Folic acid, *x*, 12, 31, 322
Fontanelle, 291, 301, 302
Food and Drug Administration
   (FDA), 13, 16
Food pyramid, *14*, 15, *289*
Food requirements, 11–15, 289
Foot-first birth, 106, 231–32, 262
Forbes, 137
Forceps, 265, 272
Forgetfulness, 91–92

Formula, 48. *See also* Bottle feeding
Formula intolerance, 286
Fourth month, 113–24
Free product samples, 47, 48
Full-term pregnancy, 242
Fundal height, 90, 189, 204

G

Gall bladder disease, 187
Gastritis, 187
Gender of baby, 56, 78, 86
General anesthesia, 255
Genetic counseling, 19–21, 79, 180–81
Genetic problems, 74
Genetic testing, 180–81
German measles, 73
Gestational age, 30
Gestational diabetes, 69, 70, 71, 90,
   172, 184–87, 231, 316
Gestational trophoblastic disease
   (GTD), 184
Gingivitis, 58
Glucose, 70, 72, 184
Glucose challenge test (GCT),
   70–72
Glucose tolerance test (GTT), 70,
   72, 147, 172, 185
Glycosuria, 70
Goals, 131
Going-home outfits, 246, 247
Gonorrhea, 75
Grandparents, 54
Groin soreness, 241
Group B streptococcus (GBS), 74, 243

H

Hands, swelling of, 170, 193
Head-down position, 106, 228
Headaches, 33, 122, 170, 194
Health care providers. *See* Doctors
Health insurance. *See* Insurance
   coverage
Health problems, *x*, 2–3, 21, 180
Healthy diet, 11–15, 88, 289, 316
Heart disease, 21

Heartbeat of baby, 82–84, 90–91, 119, 221, 253, 256
Heartburn, 12, 59, 89, 116–17
Heat, 128, 147, 151
Hemoglobin, 12, 71
Hemolytic disease, 206
Hemorrhage, 107, 272, 273
Hemorrhoids, 117
Hepatitis B, 75
Herbs, 18, 36
Hiccups, 168, 243
High blood pressure, 20, 68, 69, 70, 170, 193–94, 231
High-risk pregnancies, 21, 180
HIV, 75
Home birth, 218
Home pregnancy tests, 30
Hormonal changes
    after pregnancy, 297, 305
    and emotions, 18–19
    during first month, 25–28
    and morning sickness, 35
    during second month, 58–59
    side effects of, 34, 38, 52
Hospitals
    arriving on-time, 234
    birthing room, 218–19
    childbirth classes, 210
    health provider referrals, 5
    packing for stay, 245–47
    policies of, 6–7, 225
    preregistration, 220
    rooming in, 225–26
    stay in, 268–69
    touring, 210
    visitors, 219–20, 268–69
Human chorionic gonadotropin
    (hCG), 25, 30, 35, 58, 59, 78, 181–82, 183
Human papillomavirus (HPV), 74
Husband Coached Childbirth, 209
Husbands. *See* Dads; Spouse
Hydatidiform mole, 182
Hygeia Foundation for Perinatal
    Loss, Inc., 200

Hyperactivity, 10
Hyperemesis gravidarum, 37, 187
Hyperphenylalanine, 174
Hypertension, 20, 68, 69, 70, 170, 193–94, 231
Hyperthermia, 15
Hyperthyroidism, 187, 307
Hypnobirthing, 209, 325
Hypothyroidism, 307
Hypoxia, 191

I, J
Incompetent cervix, 187–88, 196
Incontinence, 229
Indigestion, 12, 59, 89, 116–17
Induction, 244, 265–66
Inhibin-A, 78
Insurance coverage
    for classes, 207
    cost of, 49
    filing paperwork, 220
    options, 5–6, 45–46
    through work, 94–95
Intercourse, 65–66, 175, 299
Internal fetal monitor, 83, 253
International Childbirth Education
    Association (ICEA), 210
Intervention, 6, 223–24
Intimacy issues, 65–66, 175, 296, 312, 320–21
Intrapartum asphyxia, 189
Intrauterine growth retardation
    (IUGR), 9, 90, 105, 188–90
Intravenous (IV) line, 253, 256
Iron, 12, 31, 89, 103
Irritability, 148–49, 244
Jaundice, 190, 261

K
"Kangaroo care," 108
Kegel exercises, 122, 229
Kennell, John, 308
Ketones, 37, 69
Ketosis, 37, 69, 187
Kicking, 56, 118, 243

Kidneys, 69, 70
Klaus, Marshall, 308

L
La Leche League, 285, 291, 293
Labor
    coaching, 258, 259, 260
    comfort devices, 254
    contractions, 204–5
    engagement, 241
    fluids during, 221
    food during, 221
    hydrotherapy for, 258
    inducing, 244, 265–66
    length of, 234, 249, 260
    monitors during, 221
    pain relief options, 222–23, 254–57
    placental delivery, 262
    prep preferences, 221, 252–53
    preparing for, 233, 251–71
    pushing, 260–61
    relaxation techniques, 208, 209, 254
    stages of, 257–62
    see also Preterm labor
Lamaze classes, 147, 208–9, 325
Lamaze, Fernand, 208
Lanugo covering, 86, 202
Large babies, 186
Large families, 164–65
Last menstrual period (LMP), 23, 30
Lead paint, 44
LeBoyer classes, 209
LeBoyer, Frederick, 209
Leg cramps, 170–71
Leg numbness, 144, 171
Leg restlessness, 153
Ligament pain, 144, 147
Lightening, 241
Lightheadedness, 28
Linea nigra, 116
Liver disease, 174, 187
Local anesthesia, 255
Lochia discharge, 267–68, 298, 314
Low birth weight, 9, 61, 71, 92
Lunar months, 30

M

Macrosomia, 186, 249
March of Dimes, 73
Mastitis, 295
Maternal defense system, 120
Maternal-Infant Bonding, 308
Maternity clothes, 62–64, 122
Maternity leave
    end of, 318–19
    and goals, 130–32
    legalities, 126–27, 134
    options, 135
    planning, 94–95, 134–35, 248
    returning to work, 136
Meconium, 197, 241, 249
Medicaid, 46
Medical centers. *See* Birthing
    centers; Hospitals
Medical history, 2–3, 19–20
Medical tests, 29, 60, 67, 243
Medicare, 46
Medications, 16–18, 45
Medicinal substances, 18, 36
Melasma, 58
Meningitis, 74
Menstrual period, 23, 25, 30
Mercury, 88
Midwives
    communication skills, 7–8
    first visits, 28–29
    importance of, *xii*
    interviewing, 6–7
    referrals, 6
    selecting, 4
    visits with, 4, 28–33, 68
    see also Doctors
Minerals, 11–15
Mini-meals, 12, 36
Miscarriage
    and alcohol consumption, 10
    and amniocentesis, 81
    coping with, 199–200
    and CVS, 82
    fear of, 34

    in first trimester, 86
    and incompetent cervix, 188
    support for parents, 200
    trying again, 200
    warning signs, 198–99
Molar pregnancy, 182–84
"Mommy track," 129–30
Money-saving tips, 47–48
Monozygotic multiples, 98
Mood swings, 38, 52, 60–61. *See
    also* Emotions
Morning sickness
    causes of, 35
    increase in, 59
    length of, 34–35, 37
    and multiple gestation, 91, 100
    occurrence of, *x*, 28
    remedies for, 35–36
    severe cases, 33, 37, 182, 187, 199
    snacks for, 12
    waning, 89
Morula, 24
Mother's intuition, *xii*
Motherhood, 234, 307–9, 313–22
Mothers, 172
Mucus plug, 241, 242
Multigravida, 156
Multiple births, 97–112
    breastfeeding, 109–12
    chances of, 99–100
    deliveries, 101–2, 106–8
    diagnosis of, 101
    doctor visits, 101–2
    feeding, 109–12
    full terms, 102
    pregnancy symptoms, 100–101
    premature births, 102, 106–8
    problems during, 102–6
    schedules, 109
    sleep schedules, 109
    support for parents, 101, 108–9,
        325, 332
Multitasking, 51
Murkoff, Heidi, 161

N

Naming baby, 95, 237
National Association for the
    Education of Young Children
    (NAEYC), 319
Natural childbirth, 209, 223
Nausea and vomiting of pregnancy
    (NVP)
    causes of, 35
    increase in, 59
    length of, 34–35, 37
    and multiple gestation, 91, 100
    occurrence of, *x*, 28
    remedies for, 35–36
    severe cases, 33, 37, 182, 187, 199
    snacks for, 12
    waning, 89
Neonatal intensive care unit (NICU),
    108, 196
Nesting, 235–36
Neural tube defects, 12–13, 17, 31,
    78, 80, 90
*New Mothers' Guide to
    Breastfeeding, The*, 285
Nicotine replacement therapy
    (NRT), 9, 10
Ninth month, 239–50
Nipples, for bottles, 286
Nipples, inverted, 292
Nipples, sore, 279
Non-stress test (NST), 83, 84
Nuclear medicine, 128, 129
Nurseries, 40–41, 235
Nurses, 4, 6–7
Nursing. *See* Breastfeeding
Nursing bras, 203–4, 284–85
Nutrasweet, 174
Nutrition guides, 11

O

Ob-Gyn, 4, 6–7. *See also* Doctors;
    Midwives
Occupational hazards, 128
Odors, 35

Office visits. *See* Doctors
Oligohydramnios, 189, 191
Organizations, 329–31
Overdue baby, 248–49
Oxytocin, 262, 266
Oxytocin challenge test, 84

P

Packing for hospital stay, 245–47
Pampering, 173–74
Pancreatitis, 187
Pap smears, 68, 74
Paracervical block, 257
Parent-child bonding, 108
Parental touch, 108
Parenthood, 51–54
Parenting publications, 47
Partner
   doctor visits, 29
   pregnancy symptoms, 52, 66
   role of, 38, 95–96, 123–24, 249–50
   sexual intimacy with, 65–66, 175, 296, 312
   sharing pregnancy with, 51–52
   see also Dads
Paternity leave, 126, 127, 134, 138
Patience, *xi*, 234
Pavlov, Ivan, 208
Pediatrician, 211
Pelvic exams, 68, 74
Pelvic inflammatory disease (PID), 181
Pelvic tilt exercises, 144, *145*
Perinatologist, 4, 79, 81, 101–2, 180
Perineal area, soothing, 267, 298
Pets, 310
Phenylketonuria (PKU), 174
Phone calls, 7, 32–33
Picture taking, 219
Pitocin, 84, 262, 266
Placenta, 86, 115, 190
Placental abruption, 9, 106, 192
Placental accreta, 192–93
Placental delivery, 262
Placental membranes, 24
Placental previa, 9, 65, 106, 191–92

Placental problems, 20, 106, 190–93, 231
Playgroups, 53–54
Pneumonia, 74
Polymerase chain reaction (PCR) test, 75
Post-term baby, 248–49
Postpartum depression, 305–7
Postpartum events, 298–99
Postpartum hemorrhage, 107, 273
Postpartum planning, 226
Postpartum psychosis, 306
Preeclampsia, 68, 69, 70, 104, 170, 183, 193–94
Pregnancy announcements, 93–95, 128–29
Pregnancy checklist, 341–44
Pregnancy confirmation, 30
Pregnancy Discrimination Act, 126–27
Pregnancy, enjoying, 173–75
Pregnancy induced hypertension (PIH), 193–94
Pregnancy information, 323–32
Pregnancy Labeling Task Force, 16
Pregnancy, length of, 30
Pregnancy symptoms
   first trimester, 27–28, 59, 89, 91–92, 100–101
   second trimester, 115–18, 147, 170–72
   third trimester, 204–5, 230–31, 241
Premature births
   growth following, 318
   and intensive care, 108
   of multiples, 102, 106–8
   problems during, 106–7
   risk for, 188, 194–95
   and smoking, 9
   support for parents, 108–9
   weight gains, 108
Premature dilation, 65, 187–88
Premature rupture of membranes (PROM), 9, 104, 195, 196
Prenatal care costs, 45
Prenatal care visit, 28–29
Prenatal complications, 9

Prenatal vitamins, 31, 36, 316
Preparations, *x*, 1–21, 245–48
Preregistration, 220
Prescription drugs, 16
Preterm dilation, 103
Preterm labor
   and intercourse, 65
   and multiple births, 102, 103
   risk for, 194–96, 231
   and stress, 61
   testing for, 80
   treatment, 195–96
   warning signs, 195
Progesterone, 25, 27, 58
Projectile vomiting, 286
Protein, 69–70, 78, 170, 194
Psychoprophylaxis, 208
Psychosocial problems, 9
Ptyalism, 34
Pudendal block, 257
Puffiness, 33, 170, 230

Q

Quadruplets. *See* Multiple gestation
Queasiness, 28, 37. *See also* Morning sickness
Quickening, 56, 118

R

Racial heritage, 2
Radiation exposure, 128, 129
Readiness, 1–21
Recommended Daily Allowance (RDA), 11, 13–14, 289
Regional anesthesia, 255
Registered nurse (RN), 4
Religious backgrounds, 54
Renal impairment, 69
Repetitive movement, 128
Respiratory distress syndrome (RDS), 106–7
Rest, 196–98. *See also* Sleep requirements
Restless leg syndrome (RLS), 153
Retardation, 10, 11

Retroverted uterus, 82, 91
Rh factor, 72, 80, 206
Rh immune globulin (RhoGAM), 206
Rhesus, 72
RhoGAM, 73
Round ligament pain, 144, 147
Rubella, 73

S

Saddle block, 257
Safety at home, 41
Saliva, excessive, 34, 36, 59
Sanitary pads, 267
Savings, 49–50
Sciatica, 171
Screening tests, 29, 60, 67, 243
Seat belts, 42, 171
Second-hand smoke, 44, 128, 176
Second month, 55–66
Second pregnancies, 155–65
Second-time parents, 51
Second trimester
    emotions during, 123–24, 148–49
    symptoms during, 115–18, 147, 170–72
    weight gain during, 116, 170, 194
Separation anxieties, 136
Seventh month, 201–13
Sexual intimacy, 65–66, 175, 296, 312, 320–21
Sexually transmitted diseases (STDs), 73, 74, 75
Shock, 192
Shoulder pain, 182
Siblings
    classes for, 211
    involving, 162–63, 310–11
    with new baby, 158–63
    and pregnancy, 161
    regressions, 162
    rivalry, 51, 160, 310
Sickle cell anemia, 73, 181, 231
Single mothers, 52–53, 332
Sitz bath, 268
Sixth month, 167–77
Skin pigmentation, 58

Skin-to-skin contact, 108
Sleep deprivation, 141, 149–50
Sleep positions
    for baby, 40, 304
    during pregnancy, 150–51
Sleep requirements
    after birth, 235, 308, 317
    for baby, 109, 304
    enhancing sleep patterns, 150–52
    during pregnancy, 27, 149–50
Smoking
    after birth, 317
    cost of, 9
    in first trimester, 9–10
    quitting, 9–10
    risk of, x, 9, 194
    second-hand smoke, 44, 128, 176
Snacks, 12
Snoring, 151
Sonogram, 75–78. See also
    Ultrasounds
Special-needs newborn, 21
Speculum, 68
Spider veins, 143
Spinal bifida, 12
Spinal block, 257, 263
Sports, 15, 122
Spotting, 27, 32. See also Vaginal
    discharge
Spouse
    doctor visits, 29
    pregnancy symptoms, 52, 66
    role of, 38, 95–96, 123–24, 249–50
    sexual intimacy with, 65–66, 175, 296, 312, 320–21
    sharing pregnancy with, 51–52
    see also Dads
Standing, 128
State Children's Health Insurance
    Program (SCHIP), 46
Stem cells, 262
Stepsiblings, 159
Stillbirths, 9
Stress
    on breastfeeding, 292

on dads, 177
    effects of, x, 19, 61–62
    managing, 62, 134, 149, 173, 174, 234
Stress test, 84
Stretch marks, 143–44, 314
Striae gravidarum, 143–44
Substance abuse, 9, 16
Sudden infant death syndrome
    (SIDS), 9, 40, 304
Supplements, 12–13, 16, 35–36
Swelling, of body, 33
Swelling, of feet, 122, 169–70, 193
Sympathy pains, 52, 66
Synthetic estrogen, 188
Syphilis, 75

T

Tandem nursing, 110
Tay-Sachs disease, 181
Telecommuting, 131, 138
Telemetry, 83, 253
Teratogen exposure, 17, 128
Tests. See Diagnostic tests
Thalassemia, 73
Third month, 85–96
Third trimester
    emotions during, 234, 243–44
    symptoms during, 204–5, 230–31, 241
    weight gain during, 229, 241
Thyroid problems, 187, 306–7
Tilted uterus, 82, 91
Tiredness, 27, 59
Tocolytic drugs, 104, 107, 195
Toxemia, 69, 170, 183, 193–94. See
    also Preeclampsia
Toxoplasmosis, 59
Transabdominal ultrasound, 75–78, 80, 84, 90
Transvaginal ultrasound, 75–76
Travel concerns, 42, 171, 231
Triplets. See Multiple gestation
Trisomies, 78, 181, 182

Twins
chances of, 99–100
fertilization of, *98*
fraternal twins, 98, 99
full terms, 102
identical twins, 98
and morning sickness, 91
problems faced, 104–6
see also Multiple gestation

U

Ultrasounds, 75–78, 80, 84, 90
Umbilical cord
banking, 262
care of, 303
cutting, 224–25, 261
development of, 56
entanglement, 104, 106, 115
Underdevelopment, 10, 11
United States Department of
Agriculture (USDA), 15
Urinary tract infection (UTI), 69, 71
Urination, 27, 33, 59, 229, 242
Urine tests, 29, 30, 68–69
Uterine infection, 81
Uteroplacental insufficiency (UPI), 191
Uterus
implantation in, 24
measuring, 90, 189
size of, 116, 204, 298
tilted uterus, 82, 91
top of, 90

V

Vacuum extraction, 273
Vaginal birth after cesarean (VBAC),
156–57, 210, 272
Vaginal bleeding, 122, 144, 182, 183,
188, 191–92, 195, 198
Vaginal delivery
after cesarean sections, 156–57,
210
for breech births, 231–32
moment of, 260–61
for multiple births, 106

Vaginal discharge, 27, 32, 59, 195,
197, 199, 205
Vaginal infections, 196
Vaginal secretions, 26–27
Vanishing twin syndrome, 105
Varicella infection, 73, 119
Varicose veins, 143
Vehicle safety, 41–42, 171
Vernix caseosa, 143
Vertex position, 106, 228
Videotaping, 219, 224
Vision problems, 33, 122, 170, 194,
230, 231
Vitamins, 11–15, 31, 36, 316
Vomiting. *See* Morning sickness

W

"Water breaking," 242
Water, drinking, 102, 117, 289, 299,
316
Water retention, 170, 230
Weight gain
breakdown of, 88–89
excessive weight gain, 170
first trimester, 58, 87
individuality of, 92
second trimester, 116
slowdown in, 229, 241
stretch marks, 143–44
sudden weight gain, 194
third trimester, 229, 241
Weight lifting, 128
Weight loss
of baby, 300
of mother, 187, 290, 314, 322
*What to Expect When Mommy's
Having a Baby*, 161
Wine, 10–11
Womanly Art of Breastfeeding, The,
285
Womb. *See* Uterus
Women, Infants, and Children
(WIC) program, 46, 47, 53
Work issues, 125–40, 248, 278,
318–19

Worker's Compensation laws, 127
Working Mother, 137

X, Y, Z

X-rays, 128, 129
Yolk sac, 25
Zygote, 24

THE EVERYTHING PREGNANCY ORGANIZER

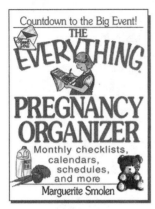

Spiral bound paperback
$15.00 ($22.95 CAN)
1-58062-336-0, 336 pages

By Marguerite Smolen

*T*he *Everything® Pregnancy Organizer* features everything a mother-to-be needs to get ready for a new baby. Complete with dozens of worksheets, checklists, pockets, and loads of helpful hints, this handy planner can help organize every aspect of your pregnancy. Arranged in an easy-to-use, month-by-month format, *The Everything® Pregnancy Organizer* is a calendar, journal, and medical resource. From keeping track of doctors' appointments and medical test results to creating shopping lists and choosing the perfect name, this organizer can become an expectant mom's best friend.

OTHER *EVERYTHING®* BOOKS BY ADAMS MEDIA CORPORATION

BUSINESS

Everything® **Business Planning Book**
Everything® **Coaching and Mentoring Book**
Everything® **Fundraising Book**
Everything® **Home-Based Business Book**
Everything® **Leadership Book**
Everything® **Managing People Book**
Everything® **Network Marketing Book**
Everything® **Online Business Book**
Everything® **Project Management Book**
Everything® **Selling Book**
Everything® **Start Your Own Business Book**
Everything® **Time Management Book**

COMPUTERS

Everything® **Build Your Own Home Page Book**

Everything® **Computer Book**
Everything® **Internet Book**
Everything® **Microsoft® Word 2000 Book**

COOKBOOKS

Everything® **Barbecue Cookbook**
Everything® **Bartender's Book, $9.95**
Everything® **Chinese Cookbook**
Everything® **Chocolate Cookbook**
Everything® **Cookbook**
Everything® **Dessert Cookbook**
Everything® **Diabetes Cookbook**
Everything® **Low-Carb Cookbook**
Everything® **Low-Fat High-Flavor Cookbook**
Everything® **Mediterranean Cookbook**
Everything® **Mexican Cookbook**
Everything® **One-Pot Cookbook**
Everything® **Pasta Book**

Everything® **Quick Meals Cookbook**
Everything® **Slow Cooker Cookbook**
Everything® **Soup Cookbook**
Everything® **Thai Cookbook**
Everything® **Vegetarian Cookbook**
Everything® **Wine Book**

HEALTH

Everything® **Anti-Aging Book**
Everything® **Diabetes Book**
Everything® **Dieting Book**
Everything® **Herbal Remedies Book**
Everything® **Hypnosis Book**
Everything® **Menopause Book**
Everything® **Nutrition Book**
Everything® **Reflexology Book**
Everything® **Stress Management Book**
Everything®**Vitamins, Minerals, and Nutritional Supplements Book**

All Everything® books are priced at $12.95 or $14.95, unless otherwise stated. Prices subject to change without notice.
Canadian prices range from $11.95–$31.95, and are subject to change without notice.

HISTORY

Everything® **American History Book**
Everything® **Civil War Book**
Everything® **Irish History & Heritage Book**
Everything® **Mafia Book**
Everything® **World War II Book**

HOBBIES & GAMES

Everything® **Bridge Book**
Everything® **Candlemaking Book**
Everything® **Casino Gambling Book**
Everything® **Chess Basics Book**
Everything® **Collectibles Book**
Everything® **Crossword and Puzzle Book**
Everything® **Digital Photography Book**
Everything® **Family Tree Book**
Everything® **Games Book**
Everything® **Knitting Book**
Everything® **Magic Book**
Everything® **Motorcycle Book**
Everything® **Online Genealogy Book**
Everything® **Photography Book**
Everything® **Pool & Billiards Book**
Everything® **Quilting Book**
Everything® **Scrapbooking Book**
Everything® **Soapmaking Book**

HOME IMPROVEMENT

Everything® **Feng Shui Book**
Everything® **Gardening Book**
Everything® **Home Decorating Book**
Everything® **Landscaping Book**
Everything® **Lawn Care Book**
Everything® **Organize Your Home Book**

KIDS' STORY BOOKS

Everything® **Bedtime Story Book**
Everything® **Bible Stories Book**
Everything® **Fairy Tales Book**
Everything® **Mother Goose Book**

EVERYTHING® *KIDS'* BOOKS

All titles are $6.95
Everything® **Kids' Baseball Book, 2nd Ed.** ($10.95 CAN)
Everything® **Kids' Bugs Book** ($10.95 CAN)
Everything® **Kids' Christmas Puzzle & Activity Book** ($10.95 CAN)
Everything® **Kids' Cookbook** ($10.95 CAN)
Everything® **Kids' Halloween Puzzle & Activity Book** ($10.95 CAN)
Everything® **Kids' Joke Book** ($10.95 CAN)
Everything® **Kids' Math Puzzles Book** ($10.95 CAN)
Everything® **Kids' Mazes Book** ($10.95 CAN)
Everything® **Kids' Money Book** ($11.95 CAN)
Everything® **Kids' Monsters Book** ($10.95 CAN)
Everything® **Kids' Nature Book** ($11.95 CAN)
Everything® **Kids' Puzzle Book** ($10.95 CAN)
Everything® **Kids' Science Experiments Book** ($10.95 CAN)
Everything® **Kids' Soccer Book** ($10.95 CAN)
Everything® **Kids' Travel Activity Book** ($10.95 CAN)

LANGUAGE

Everything® **Learning French Book**
Everything® **Learning German Book**
Everything® **Learning Italian Book**
Everything® **Learning Latin Book**
Everything® **Learning Spanish Book**
Everything® **Sign Language Book**

MUSIC

Everything® **Drums Book (with CD)**, $19.95 ($31.95 CAN)
Everything® **Guitar Book**
Everything® **Playing Piano and Keyboards Book**

Everything® **Rock & Blues Guitar Book (with CD)**, $19.95 ($31.95 CAN)
Everything® **Songwriting Book**

NEW AGE

Everything® **Astrology Book**
Everything® **Divining the Future Book**
Everything® **Dreams Book**
Everything® **Ghost Book**
Everything® **Meditation Book**
Everything® **Numerology Book**
Everything® **Palmistry Book**
Everything® **Psychic Book**
Everything® **Spells & Charms Book**
Everything® **Tarot Book**
Everything® **Wicca and Witchcraft Book**

PARENTING

Everything® **Baby Names Book**
Everything® **Baby Shower Book**
Everything® **Baby's First Food Book**
Everything® **Baby's First Year Book**
Everything® **Breastfeeding Book**
Everything® **Father-to-Be Book**
Everything® **Get Ready for Baby Book**
Everything® **Homeschooling Book**
Everything® **Parent's Guide to Positive Discipline**
Everything® **Potty Training Book**, $9.95 ($15.95 CAN)
Everything® **Pregnancy Book, 2nd Ed.**
Everything® **Pregnancy Fitness Book**
Everything® **Pregnancy Organizer**, $15.00 ($22.95 CAN)
Everything® **Toddler Book**
Everything® **Tween Book**

PERSONAL FINANCE

Everything® **Budgeting Book**
Everything® **Get Out of Debt Book**
Everything® **Get Rich Book**
Everything® **Homebuying Book, 2nd Ed.**
Everything® **Homeselling Book**

All Everything® books are priced at $12.95 or $14.95, unless otherwise stated. Prices subject to change without notice.
Canadian prices range from $11.95–$31.95, and are subject to change without notice.

Everything® **Investing Book**
Everything® **Money Book**
Everything® **Mutual Funds Book**
Everything® **Online Investing Book**
Everything® **Personal Finance Book**
Everything® **Personal Finance in Your 20s & 30s Book**
Everything® **Wills & Estate Planning Book**

PETS

Everything® **Cat Book**
Everything® **Dog Book**
Everything® **Dog Training and Tricks Book**
Everything® **Horse Book**
Everything® **Puppy Book**
Everything® **Tropical Fish Book**

REFERENCE

Everything® **Astronomy Book**
Everything® **Car Care Book**
Everything® **Christmas Book, $15.00** ($21.95 CAN)
Everything® **Classical Mythology Book**
Everything® **Einstein Book**
Everything® **Etiquette Book**
Everything® **Great Thinkers Book**
Everything® **Philosophy Book**
Everything® **Shakespeare Book**
Everything® **Tall Tales, Legends, & Other Outrageous Lies Book**
Everything® **Toasts Book**
Everything® **Trivia Book**
Everything® **Weather Book**

RELIGION

Everything® **Angels Book**
Everything® **Buddhism Book**
Everything® **Catholicism Book**
Everything® **Jewish History & Heritage Book**
Everything® **Judaism Book**

Everything® **Prayer Book**
Everything® **Saints Book**
Everything® **Understanding Islam Book**
Everything® **World's Religions Book**
Everything® **Zen Book**

SCHOOL & CAREERS

Everything® **After College Book**
Everything® **College Survival Book**
Everything® **Cover Letter Book**
Everything® **Get-a-Job Book**
Everything® **Hot Careers Book**
Everything® **Job Interview Book**
Everything® **Online Job Search Book**
Everything® **Resume Book, 2nd Ed.**
Everything® **Study Book**

SELF-HELP

Everything® **Dating Book**
Everything® **Divorce Book**
Everything® **Great Marriage Book**
Everything® **Great Sex Book**
Everything® **Romance Book**
Everything® **Self-Esteem Book**
Everything® **Success Book**

SPORTS & FITNESS

Everything® **Bicycle Book**
Everything® **Body Shaping Book**
Everything® **Fishing Book**
Everything® **Fly-Fishing Book**
Everything® **Golf Book**
Everything® **Golf Instruction Book**
Everything® **Pilates Book**
Everything® **Running Book**
Everything® **Sailing Book, 2nd Ed.**
Everything® **T'ai Chi and QiGong Book**
Everything® **Total Fitness Book**
Everything® **Weight Training Book**
Everything® **Yoga Book**

TRAVEL

Everything® **Guide to Las Vegas**

Everything® **Guide to New England**
Everything® **Guide to New York City**
Everything® **Guide to Washington D.C.**
Everything® **Travel Guide to The Disneyland Resort®, California Adventure®, Universal Studios®, and the Anaheim Area**
Everything® **Travel Guide to the Walt Disney World Resort®, Universal Studios®, and Greater Orlando, 3rd Ed.**

WEDDINGS

Everything® **Bachelorette Party Book**
Everything® **Bridesmaid Book**
Everything® **Creative Wedding Ideas Book**
Everything® **Jewish Wedding Book**
Everything® **Wedding Book, 2nd Ed.**
Everything® **Wedding Checklist, $7.95** ($11.95 CAN)
Everything® **Wedding Etiquette Book, $7.95** ($11.95 CAN)
Everything® **Wedding Organizer, $15.00** ($22.95 CAN)
Everything® **Wedding Shower Book, $7.95** ($12.95 CAN)
Everything® **Wedding Vows Book, $7.95** ($11.95 CAN)
Everything® **Weddings on a Budget Book, $9.95** ($15.95 CAN)

WRITING

Everything® **Creative Writing Book**
Everything® **Get Published Book**
Everything® **Grammar and Style Book**
Everything® **Grant Writing Book**
Everything® **Guide to Writing Children's Books**
Everything® **Screenwriting Book**
Everything® **Writing Well Book**